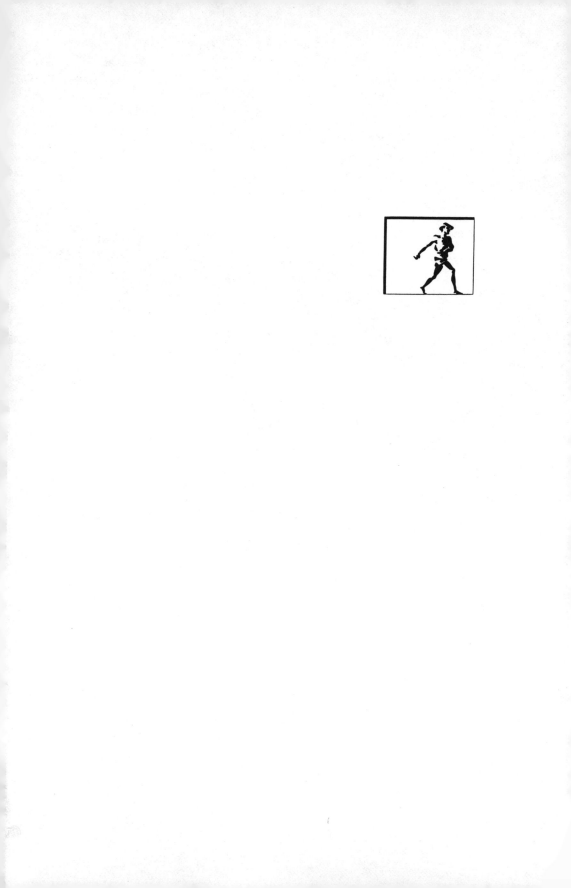

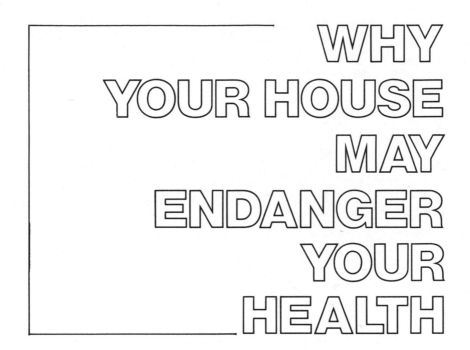

WHY YOUR HOUSE MAY ENDANGER YOUR HEALTH

Alfred V. Zamm, M.D., F.A.C.A., F.A.C.P.
with Robert Gannon

SIMON AND SCHUSTER

NEW YORK

Published by Simon and Schuster
A Division of Gulf & Western Corporation
Simon & Schuster Building
Rockefeller Center
1230 Avenue of the Americas
New York, New York 10020

SIMON AND SCHUSTER and colophon are trademarks of
Simon & Schuster

Designed by Stanley S. Drate

Manufactured in the United States of America

1 2 3 4 5 6 7 8 9 10

Library of Congress Cataloging in Publication Data

Zamm, Alfred V
    Why your house may endanger your health.

    Includes bibliographical references and index.
    1. Housing and health.   2. Environmentally induced
diseases.   3. Dwellings—Environmental engineering.
I. Gannon, Robert, joint author.   II. Title.
RA770.Z34   616.9′8   80-12277
ISBN 0-671-24128-1

The authors gratefully acknowledge permission to reprint excerpts from the following:

"Human Sensitivity to Electric Fields," by Clarence W. Wieska in *Biomedical Sciences Instrumentation,* Vol. 1 (1963), pp. 467–74, copyright © 1963 Instrument Society of America.
"Ruminations: The Great Winds of the Earth," by Robert H. Moser in *Journal of the American Medical Association,* Vol. 227, No. 2 (January 14, 1974), pp. 195–96, copyright © 1974 American Medical Association.
Speech by Theron G. Randolph, M.D., reprinted in *Human Ecology Study Group Bulletin,* Summer, 1977. Reprinted by permission.
Letter from Norman Rafalowsky to editor of *The Daily Freeman,* Kingston, N.Y., January 8, 1976. Reprinted by permission.

To my wife, Marlane
A.V.Z.

_____ Acknowledgments

Any book requires the help of a great many people—this one more than most, because the research resulted not only in a book, but in the building of a prototype healthy house. Among the many to whom the debt extends, the following were especially helpful:

Dorothy Dolce (Kingston, NY), librarian; Samuel Liebman and Joseph Hurwitz (New Paltz, NY), design and architecture; Thomas Ryan and David Biggs (Troy, NY), structural engineering; Goldman, Sokolow & Copeland (New York, NY), mechanical engineering; Robert Cross (Bearsville, NY), site engineering, surveying, and source of solid, practical ideas; Albert Pray (Lake Hill, NY), poured concrete foundation; Fred DeVito and James Purcell (Schenectady, NY), masonry/block work; Ulisse Marchette (Hurley, NY), masonry/block work; Donald and Jack Schoonmaker (Kingston, NY), carpentry; John Kuriplach (Saugerties, NY), roofing; Harry Wiands and George Lent (Kingston, NY), electrical; Stuart Smedes and crew (Kingston, NY), plumbing; Aaron Van deBogart (Bearsville, NY), earthmoving; Fred Shader (Woodstock, NY), earthmoving; Lynn Barry and Judith Klugman, research; Cherene Holland, editorial guidance through various stages of the manuscript; Frederic W. Hills, Simon and Schuster Senior Editor.

Information about commerical products and industrial processes often is obtainable only from people with great experience in the field. No amount of library research can replace experience. The following companies were helpful in the development of some of the ideas in this book, and their products and services were used to build the house based upon this book:

D'Agostino Building Blocks, Inc. (1111 Altamour Ave., Schenectady, NY 12303), exterior veneer block; Structural Stoneware, Inc. (P.O. Box 119, Minerva, OH 44657), tile floor; Elon, Inc. (964 Third Ave., New York, NY 10022), tiles; The Briare Co., Inc. (775 Brooklyn Ave., Baldwin, NY 11510), bathroom tiles; Pratt & Lambert (P.O. Box 22, Buffalo, NY 14240), interior paint and alkyd paint; West Rock Electric Corp. (396 Ashford Ave., Dobbs Ferry, NY 10522), vacuum system installation; George Kovacs, Inc. (831 Madison Ave., New York, NY 10021), lighting; Habitat, Inc. (150 E. 58th St., New York, NY 10021), lighting; Koch & Lowy (940 Third Ave., New York, NY 10022), lighting; Victor Mfg. Co. (1045 Terminal Way, San Carlos, CA 94070), lighting; Design Research International, Inc. (48 Brattle St., Cambridge, MA 02138), furniture; Brown Jorden (9860 Gidley St., P.O. Box 1269, El Monte, CA 91734), outdoor furniture; NuTone Div. of Scovill Co. (Madison & Redbank Rds., Cincinnati, OH 45227), miscellaneous electrical appliances; Iron-A-Way Co., Inc. (220 W. Jackson St., Morton, IL 61550), ironing board (convertible, folding); Kitchen-Aid Division, Hobart Corp. (Troy, OH 45374), kitchen appliances; Bogen Division, Lear Siegler, Inc. (P.O. Box 500, Paramus, NJ 07652), intercom system (All-Master stations; model #LI-7A); Motorola, Communications & Electronics, Inc. (1301 E. Algonquin Road, Schaumburg, IL 60196), communications systems; Arneson Products (P.O. Box 2009, Koch Road, Corte Madera, CA 94925), pool cleaning equipment ("Pool Sweep"); Onan Corporation (1400 73rd Ave. N.E., Minneapolis, MN 55432), design of minimal-pollution propane standby electric generator.

Research for this book was supported in part by a grant from the Liberal Arts College Fund for Research, The Pennsylvania State University.

Contents

_____ Preface

Few people know that the air inside the average American home is more polluted than that outside. Fewer still are aware that allergic reactions now constitute the single greatest source of illness in Western society. Or that the electricity in our homes can change our moods and affect our cells. Or that the common household chemicals present in nearly every home—cleaners, waxes, polishes, heating fuels—can bring about illness without ever revealing themselves as the cause. And almost nobody realizes that we can become addicted to the very toxic substances that are making us ill.

The degree to which a person recognizes those forces places him in one of three categories:

1. He is an environmentally sensitive individual, and he knows it. He may react adversely to housedust and certain fumes, for example, and he has learned to avoid those conditions that will make him sick.

2. He is extremely sensitive and does _not_ know it—depressed much of the time, tired without good reason, weak and logy and slow-thinking. But he has adapted, and he may even think that such a state is _natural_.

3. Or he is apparently unaffected by his environment. And yet, surrounded by incipient poisons, he may not be —_probably_ isn't—reaching his potential. Because the fact is, everyone is environmentally susceptible to some degree.

This book tries to bring about an awareness of the household entities that may cause problems—to examine living habits, then to suggest simple alternatives in living habits. It is divided into three general parts. The first shows what the average home is like, shows the myriad common substances that to one extent or another are unhealthful, and surveys the symptoms that an unhealthy environment can bring about. The second part discusses what to do about it—what products to use, what clothing and furnishings to buy, and the best way to maintain a home for the well-being of those who live there. The third part is designed for the person who is considering moving to a new home, renovating his present one, or building a new one. It shows where to live, the kind of house one should select, and the components to be incorporated in the design. An appendix is also provided to help the homeowner find out if he is being affected by his surroundings.

Our concern here is not necessarily with the chemically sensitive person who knows he *must* make certain changes in his environment, but with the vast majority who don't even realize that their surroundings are making life a little more difficult than it should be. And possibly a bit shorter.

Introduction

In the last quarter of the twentieth century, man suddenly finds himself living on an alien planet. He hasn't been there before, and his body doesn't know how to adapt. Since he first appeared on earth, he's gone through something like 175,000 generations—and all of them, until recently, ate generally the same kind of food, drank the same water, breathed the same air. Now all of this has changed. His food has altered dramatically. His water contains hitherto unencountered chemicals. And his shelter, his home, is no longer *natural*, but is filled with new forces acting upon him: strange vapors, foreign particles, alien electromagnetic energy. In only a sliver of evolutionary time, man has drastically transformed the world.

For nearly all of the three or four million years that man has been around, his habitat, the earth, has been relatively stable. Over the eons the air makeup changed somewhat (as he learned to breathe smoke from campfires), and his food supply and eating habits altered a bit (a result of farming, invented some 10,000 years ago), but the changes were comparatively moderate, and because they happened over thousands of years, the human body was able to accept them with relative ease. The biggest variation was in climate—but man's brain allowed him to fashion shelters to modify harsh weather.

Natural selection shaped our ancestors to make them superbly able to deal with their environment. Over the last half century or so, however, two things have happened to change that environment. First, the world has experienced a chemical avalanche. And second, man has polluted his air, his water, his food. And now the environment is striking back in ways we have only begun to grasp. The human being is an accommodating animal, but evolution is slow, and the environmental changes are occurring much faster than man can adapt.

The precise effect of this alien environment is unclear —it can't even be measured yet—but its results are increasingly becoming apparent. And they are profound. Says Dr. John Knowles, president of the Rockefeller Foundation: "Over 99 percent of us are born healthy and made sick as a result of personal misbehavior and environmental conditions."[1]

In modern-day America, a new compound is synthesized and added to the environment at the rate of one a *minute*. Nobody knows what the total is, but the American Chemical Society's computerized registry, the *Chemical Abstracts Service,* now lists more than four *million* entries (most of them developed only recently), with an estimated 63,000 thought to be in common use in this country.[2] This proliferation of never-before-seen chemicals is so out of control as to be stunning. Society can outlaw the most hazardous, but with a quarter million new substances entering the world every year, nobody can keep track of what they really are, what they can do, what they might do to the environment. The result: We are immersed in a strange chemical ocean, an ocean that has existed for only a moment in the earth's history.

To put the time in perspective, think of man's history in terms of distance. If his whole stay on earth stretches from Los Angeles to New York City, the chemical revolution occupies only the last 211 feet. Or look at it this way: If man has been on earth the equivalent of one full year, he's been surrounded by this drastically altered environment during only the last 7.5 minutes. That's a powerful jolt for an individual, and an equally massive shock for a species. In the history of the world thousands of species have been wiped out because of changes not nearly so profound.

One person who has a good grasp of the fragility of life is anthropologist Richard Leakey, and he, too, fears the ever-more-hostile environment that man is creating for himself. "People feel that we are here by predestination and that because we are humans we will be able to survive even if we make mistakes," Leakey told a reporter from *Time* magazine in 1977. He added that few people understand that the human being is simply another organism. "There have been thousands of living organisms, of which a very high percentage has become extinct," he said. "There is nothing, at the moment, to suggest that we are not part of that same pattern." But man is the only species with power to reflect on its past and upon its future, and to see the changes taking place. Said Leakey, with only a hint of optimism: "We have the power that makes it possible to plan our future in such a way as to avoid what seems inevitable."[3]

Most scientists don't take such a negative view; few, in fact, feel that *Homo sapiens* is anywhere near being wiped out. But those who have looked into the situation have little doubt that as individuals, human beings have some very rough times ahead—and a great many people are going through day-to-day hell right now without the foggiest notion as to why, without even an inkling that their problems are being caused by their environment, by foreign entities never before experienced in the history of man.

Each new alien substance the body's cells have to adjust to requires energy, the cumulative effect of which is labeled *stress*. The cell, the body, the man, can't indefinitely maintain adaption under stress. Eventually, barring other calamities, virtually every heavy smoker will die from a smoking-induced illness. And although the woman who, every few days, breathes acetone from nail-polish remover probably won't die from that, when coupled with the hundreds of other chemicals that daily assault her system, the acetone might very well push her over the edge into episodes of "unexplained" depression.

The answer, of course, is to avoid as many alien chemicals as possible, to protect the cell from as many blows as possible so that it isn't overwhelmed, to remove as many foreign substances from the environment as possible, to protect the cell by sheltering it. What man has been doing for the past million years or so is building a shelter for himself—a shelter for his body in the form of a home, a shelter for his cells in the form of a body. And that's what this book is all about. Shelters. Houses. Healthy ones.

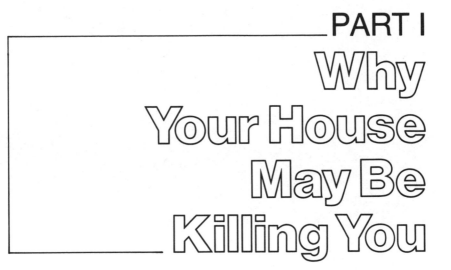

PART I

Why Your House May Be Killing You

1

Why Worry?

The idea that people can be made sick by harmful substances certainly isn't new. You eat something that doesn't agree with you and you get a stomachache; you select the wrong kind of deodorant and break out in an underarm rash; you spend an evening in a smoke-filled room and get a headache. Nothing astounding there. The thing that is surprising is the *magnitude* of it all—something physicians are just beginning to realize.

The medical profession today is on the threshold of a revolution, one comparable to that caused by Pasteur's discovery that infectious diseases are the result of toxins produced by specific microbes. Medicine, for the past hundred years, has concentrated almost exclusively on these microbes—with admittedly spectacular results. Man no longer experiences devastating epidemics of such infectious diseases as cholera, smallpox, tuberculosis, and typhoid. But he suffers less dramatic but more insidious epidemics of high blood pressure, stroke, heart disease, bowel problems, cancer, obesity, allergy, and a barrage of mental illnesses.

One reason the incidence of these nonmicrobial diseases has risen is that we're living longer. Penicillin and its descendants have virtually wiped out the big killers of the last century. But that isn't the whole story. With increasing clarity the world's physicians—particularly those specializing in cellular physiology—are seeing that the major cause of twentieth-century disease is what we've done to our food, water, and air. We're surrounded by the disease of industrialism.

The study of these environmental causes of disease can be placed in a new branch of medicine—still controversial and relatively unknown—called *clinical ecology*. It deals simply with illnesses caused by inanimate elements in the environment—particles, vapors, electrical entities—that somehow find their way into the body. The physicians who are working in this area are convinced that the real causes of many illnesses are never found because they're incorrectly diagnosed. One reason is that people with an environmental sickness may not immediately see symptoms. For example, a man might breathe aftershave fumes before breakfast, then feel depressed in the office and never relate the two, or he may be exposed to a food that gives him problems two days later. When a substance enters the body through the lungs or stomach, the bloodstream carries it to every tissue, and if the substance acts as an irritant, any area of the body can become upset. The patient, for example, may believe that his symptoms are just psychosomatic, the mind influencing the body, but what is really happening is the reverse: *somatopsychic*, the body influencing the brain.

Believing that an illness is simply psychosomatic may be a convenient way to avoid the problem, yet the patient might very well be helped, perhaps *cured,* simply by removing the offending substance from his environment: by eliminating, for example, the routine application of liquid wax to his kitchen floor every other Wednesday; the fumes from the wax, evaporating all week, might be causing him to experience constant depression.

The possibility that an unspecialized medical approach will reveal a solution is remote. Clinical ecology, although a new view of medicine, is a return to a kind of general practice, cutting across the specialties. Further, the conventional physician doesn't have the specialized training necessary to track down these answers, and *al-*

lopathic medicine, a concentration on the treatment of symptoms, may be used, because the causes are either unknown or are buried away in obscure corners of the equally obscure new specialty of ecological medicine. The clinical ecologist also treats symptoms, of course (for housedust allergy he may prescribe antihistamines), but his emphasis is on the *cause*—to try to eliminate the housedust. Some groups—the drug industry, for example, which has a stake in establishing medications as the modern solution to nearly everything—have a built-in bias toward ignoring environmental factors in disease. Many drug manufacturers, either for purposes of identification or simply to make medicines attractive, even use dyes made of coal-tar derivatives on vitamin pills prescribed for pregnant women. The artifical color has no medical value, and its effect on the fetus is unknown.

Another factor is that many physicians have a strong skepticism toward this type of environmental approach to medicine, mainly because it was not emphasized in medical schools when they got their training thirty years ago.

The big problem with tracking down such causes is that the task can be extraordinarily difficult. Medical science is still in its infancy in understanding the subtleties of how some environmental substances cause illness; there is yet no skin test or examination of blood or tissue or saliva that a physician can look at and say, "Ah, you're hypersensitive to the furniture-polish vapors you're breathing, and *that's* what's making you chemically depressed," or "That fly-killing insecticide strip hanging in the nursery is sensitizing your baby, who may face a lifetime of mental problems because of induced neurological allergy." Furthermore, there might be a considerable lag between the exposure to a harmful chemical and its effect—whether it be the chemicals breathed into the lungs from hair spray, or a food; the substance is ingested in either case.

One example of a delayed reaction is a personal story reported by Dr. Walter C. Alvarez, editor of *Modern Medicine*. For years he had experienced what he calls his

"dumb Mondays," days in which his efficiency was markedly decreased. "Every Sunday night I had much gas,
with abdominal pain and bad nightmares," he wrote in
1967. "And every Monday morning I felt so 'dumb' I
could not do much constructive work—only routine
tasks. Then I remembered that as a small boy I would
become ill if I ate chicken gravy. I quit eating my traditional chicken dinners on Sunday, and that was the end
of my 'dumb Mondays.' "[1] Surprising, yes. And the same
kind of delay can occur if the offending substance is
taken into the body as food or is breathed as a vapor or a
cloud of particles.

Still other problems take months or even years to
manifest themselves. Cigarette smokers, for example,
sometimes require half a lifetime to work up a fatal case
of cancer. Detecting a relationship between a chemical
and carcinoma is especially difficult. As was stated in
The Medical Letter in 1976:

> Relating even a moderate increase in the incidence of a
> common cancer . . . to a specific drug or other chemical
> given ten to thirty years before would be very difficult even
> in a very large study with a control group. An impression of
> safety gained through the widespread use of a drug or
> chemical, even over long periods of time, may therefore be
> misleading.[2]

Now add to that statement this comment from a *Scientific American* article: "Almost all cancers appear to be
caused by exposure to factors in the environment."[3] The
implications become truly staggering. If almost all cancers are environmentally related, and if nobody knows
what's causing them, how can we know which chemicals
to avoid?

Even if the response to an alien chemical is relatively
immediate, however, the victim might not be aware of it.
For example, there's a malady manifested by some of my
women patients that could be called the "moody mother"
syndrome: a general headachy fatigue coupled with
depression and a near claustrophobia. They feel it only at

home, particularly in their kitchens, and usually they don't bring the problem to me (at least not immediately), but to their psychiatrists. The home environment, particularly in these times of changing attitudes toward proper social roles of the sexes, can cause enormous problems for women, both emotional and physical. And many feel that because of societal suppression, of being forced into the role of wife and mother to the exclusion of everything else, women are developing emotional, psychological, or psychosomatic illnesses that don't really have organic bases, that have little to do with their surroundings—except, perhaps, symbolically. I find, however, that among many of my patients, as soon as offending substances are removed from the environment, symptoms of the "daily dismals" often leave too. If a woman who tests negatively to food and inhalants tells me that she is unhappy all of the time, *everywhere* in the house, and even on vacation, I tend to suspect that the problems may very well be strictly emotional. But as soon as she says that she gets depressed or feels fenced in only in the *kitchen,* I look to an environmental pollutant. My next question concerns her cooking range: gas or electric? A gas oven operating at 350 degrees F. for one hour, because of the inevitable incomplete combustion, can cause kitchen-air pollution —even with an exhaust fan in operation—comparable to a heavy Los Angeles smog. Without the fan, levels of carbon monoxide and nitrogen dioxide can zoom to three or more times that.[4] A great many women have become chemically sensitive to the fumes from gas stoves (after all, they may spend half their waking lives in the kitchen), and when the gas range is replaced with an electric one, the depression often disappears. Would such women benefit from psychological therapy? Certainly—if the sessions led to the decision to flee the home. But the benefit of the change would be primarily organic, not psychological.

That such fumes and other assorted chemicals are floating throughout the average home is a fact that many allergists and other clinical ecologists have known for some time. It was only a few years ago, however, that concrete statistics began to accumulate. One bit of evidence surfaced in 1976, when a team of researchers led by physician Ralph Binder of Yale University completed a study of indoor air pollution for Yale's Lung Research Center.[5] Other investigations on exposure of children to air pollution had been done before, but most of them concentrated on *outdoor* pollution. Children in the United States spend 60 to 80 percent of their time indoors, however, so the Yale group felt that measurement of indoor air was essential for the full picture. What the team did was actually very simple: sampled the air breathed by twenty high-school students for a full day. The students, ten with some evidence of respiratory problems (coughing, occasional wheezing, or a history of asthma), carried with them air samplers that ran continuously for the full time.

"At the end of the twenty-four-hour period," the team reported, "we recorded the daily activities, and details of the climatic conditions and the home environment, including the number of smokers in the home, the number of people and rooms in the home, the type of heating system used, the type of fuel used for cooking, the composition of the floors or floor coverings, the presence of open or closed windows, and the presence or absence of a fireplace and pets." When the researchers compared the results with the outdoor air samples, they were amazed to find that air in nineteen of the twenty children's homes was considerably more polluted than air outside. Concluded Binder: "Since a person's air pollutant load . . . appears to be determined primarily by indoor exposures, no significant improvement in respirable particulate loads can be expected to result from reduction of outdoor particulate levels, even in urban areas." In other words, it's not enough to filter automobile exhaust or to shut down factories with smoking chimneys if nothing is done to clean up household air.

The fact that indoor air is so much more polluted than outdoor air is not surprising when you consider all the possible sources of airborne chemicals in the home: waxes, mothballs, paint, glue, disinfectants, anything propelled by aerosols, anything that evaporates. To one extent or another, all are toxic. All you have to do is read the product labels: "Avoid prolonged contact," "Do not inhale or swallow," "Use in well-ventilated room," "Call physician immediately."

When you think about it, such chemicals, wafting throughout the house and settling in the lungs or absorbed by the bloodstream of family members, are obviously unhealthy. Other problems, however, are not so apparent. Microscopic particles stirred up by someone walking across a rug, for instance. Or low-level toxins in drinking water. Or electrical charges in the air. Or insecticide residues on (and in) fruits. Or an aerosol spray.

Such factors—the obvious and the hidden, the particles, vapors, and electrical factors—affect human beings in a whole variety of overlapping ways, but for clarification they can be classified under three headings: as *allergens,* as *toxins,* or as *subtoxins.*

An *allergen* causes an allergy (more fully discussed in Chapter 2), a heightened sensitivity to normally *harmless* substances. What happens is that the allergen enters the body by being breathed or eaten or rubbed on, and the system of the person allergic to it makes a dreadful mistake: It erroneously recognizes the allergen as an enemy and reacts by attacking it with defensive chemicals and cells. The battle profoundly affects various organs, and the result may be sneezing, itching, stomach cramps, or even, if the organ affected is the brain, psychological disturbances. What bothers an allergic person will not affect a nonallergic person, since the allergen is not harmful in itself.

For years the medical establishment estimated that one in seven adults had some sort of allergy problem. In the last decade or two, however, this has been broadened. Now the accepted ratio is one in three; one-third of all Americans show allergic symptoms sometime in their lives.[6] Both figures are probably low. Evidence is now coming to light that allergies cause many more problems than have even been contemplated: mental illness, for example, ranging all the way from mild aggression to psychosis. Some physicians are now saying that half the adult population suffers from allergies, and a few individuals are speculating that nearly *everybody,* to one extent or another, suffers from some sort of allergy. In fact, Dr. Donald McKaba, chairman of the Public Relations Committee of the American Academy of Allergy, says that allergies are the nation's number one cause of chronic illness.[7] And English physician Richard Mackarness goes even further. He says that allergy has overtaken infection to become "the number one cause of illness in Westernized society."[8]

Toxins differ from allergens in that they are intrinsic poisons that do primary damage to known metabolic areas. They're easily understood and relatively easy to deal with. But they may or may not be apparent. The fact that lead-based paints are toxic is well publicized. Few parents nowadays would paint their baby's crib without checking the can's label. But how many people consider the fact that most copper water pipes are soldered together, with the possibility of lead leaching into the water supply, to be drunk by that same baby over the next twenty years?

Subtoxins (sublethal doses of poisons) remain most elusive. These are usually thought of as harmless, at least in small amounts (a whiff of nail-polish remover, for instance, or the odor of a newly cleaned rug), but they're not harmless to *sensitive* people, those with low levels of tolerance to alien chemicals. Everyone who puts his hands in fire gets burned, but only some people get burned when they put their hands in laundry water—those who are highly sensitive to the chemicals in the detergent. Such individuals, such "delicate" people, may simply have more critical measuring equipment. They're better detectors. Their bodies may be sensing something that may have a cumulative harmful effect on others as well. And for the rest of us, these sensitive people may be valuable—by acting as our early-warning systems, like those canaries that miners used to carry with them to detect methane.

Depending on the sensitivity of the individual, minute quantities of chemicals may be exceedingly disruptive, either producing immediate and severe reactions or—unfortunately, what is usually the case—slow, insidious, and often masked reactions. The acute reactions are obvious. If someone is particularly sensitive to, say, bus fumes, he often knows it; in a bus terminal he develops a headache. So he learns to avoid the situation. But suppose an individual is sensitive to chlorine in his drinking water. And suppose the trouble manifests itself in a way that seems illogical, that is unexpected, like depression or hyperactivity or insomnia. How is the person going to isolate the cause, particularly when the effect may not appear until the next day, and particularly since the average citizen is taking hundreds of man-made chemicals into his system daily?

The picture is confusing enough, often baffling. But there's another factor that throws the problem into total chaos: The individual's body, in learning to deal with the offending substance, may have learned to *need* the source of the trouble, may require the chemical to keep the protective mechanism going, to keep the body in a state of what it feels is "well-being," may, in fact, be *addicted* to it, and will be in great turmoil if deprived—like the alcoholic, who, waking up with a hangover, feels better after his morning drink. The term that describes aspects of this mechanism is *general adaptation syndrome,* coined by the world's acknowledged expert on stress, Hans Selye. What it means is simply that the body —more particularly, the cell—learns to adapt to a bad situation. A man, or his body, or an individual cell of his body wants things to remain the same. Changes are upsetting. They're hard to deal with. But changes *must* be dealt with in one way or another, and on the cellular level, the cell either adapts or it dies. It adapts by such means as covering itself with a protective coating (a callus or a corn), or perhaps by producing additional enzymes (to handle some alien chemical it finds itself absorbing), or by some other method. But it does deal with the outside stress, using energy to do so, until the stress goes away or until the cell adapts, at which time it arrives at *homeostasis,* a state of equilibrium.

Here are two simple illustrations: One, when coffee

prices skyrocketed in 1977, many people stopped drinking coffee cold turkey—and they developed severe headaches as a result.[9] Their bodies had learned to accept a certain level of caffeine in the blood, and when the level dropped, aching heads resulted. Treatment: a cup of coffee. And two, when a heavy smoker suddenly quits, he goes through agony—not only psychological, but physical. Cigarette smoke contains hundreds of chemicals, and the cells of a smoker's body are not only *used* to those chemicals, they need them, are addicted to them. Suddenly deprived of their every-thirty-minute fix, the cells find their homeostasis badly upset, the system has to make adjustments, resistance plummets, and the ex-smoker feels terrible for weeks, until his cellular chemistry arrives at a state of equilibrium again. In the long run, cigarette smoking, of course, is extraordinarily disruptive; but in the short run, *stopping* smoking is.

The big trouble with maintaining homeostasis under stress is that it requires energy. Each new substance the body has to identify, evaluate, and adjust to requires energy, whether the substance is an allergen, a toxin, or a subtoxin. Not only might the stress produce immediate fatigue, but the more chemicals taken in, the more adaption is needed and the more cellular energy is expended. Eventually, the cell—and ultimately, the body—is overwhelmed. The body organism simply runs out of funds, and the additional energy required to deal with the constant onslaught of new substances is so great that bankruptcy results—the body gets sick.

Housedust: It's Worse Than You Think

Each time eight-year-old Jimmy visited his grandmother, he came back sneezing and blowing his nose. His father accused the grandmother of keeping the house too cold.

Every Saturday night, just as newly married Julie was getting ready to go out with her husband, she would start to develop a mild sore throat and to sniffle—the beginnings, she thought, of a cold. Sometimes she stayed home, attempting to check whatever was wrong by going to bed.

A thirty-year-old accountant who worked out of his home seemed to be developing a cold all winter, "coming down with something," he'd say—watery eyes, scratchy throat, sneezes, coughs. Most of the time he was so uncomfortable that his work took twice as long to complete as it should have, and sometimes he felt that he just couldn't think straight.

His cold never did develop. Neither did the colds of Julie or the child. The reason: They didn't have colds at all; they were all allergic to housedust. Julie worked in an office during the week and cleaned house on Saturdays. The dust she stirred up irritated her nasal passages, giving her cold symptoms. But by Sunday morning the dust had settled again, and her symptoms had gone. Jimmy's grandmother was an immaculate housekeeper, but her heavy drapes, oriental rugs, and overstuffed furniture, difficult to clean, were repositories of dust. Jimmy, a typically active youngster, would lie on the rug, climb on the furniture, disturb the drapes—all the while inhaling dust accumulated over the years. The accountant's desk sat next to a hot-air register, and all winter long dust-laden air blew across him because somebody had long ago discarded the furnace's air filter.

Unless you live in a vacuum bottle, no matter how good a housekeeper you are, you're surrounded to one degree or another by dust. You breathe it continually. You can see it when sunlight streams through the window; without dust, the rays would be invisible. One study revealed that the average six-room home in a city or in the suburbs accumulates forty pounds of dust a year.[1] Some physicians are now viewing housedust as an "ocupational hazard" for the homemaker, both because housecleaning stirs up enormous quantities of dust, and because the housewife spends most of the time in the house, breathing it.

Housedust is composed of much more than simply dirt, as the table in this chapter shows. It's an incredibly complex mixture of bits of lint, snips of hair, particles of textiles from rugs, bedding, furniture, drapes, carpet padding, clothing, and pillows. Particularly virulent for those who are sensitive is animal *dander*—the "scurf" or minute scales of animal skin, somewhat like human dandruff—associated with animal hair and often found in housedust. It's this dander that causes most allergies to animals. Often the source is the family pet, but you don't have to have a pet or live on a farm to become sensitive. Animal hair is widely used as furniture and toy stuffing —and wool, of course, comes from fleece. (If your child exhibits allergic symptoms after being licked by a dog or cat, that's a good indication he's sensitive.)

Another villain hidden in housedust is mold, or more accurately, mold spores. In winter this is less of a problem, unless your basement is particularly damp. But in the warm months, when humidity rises, molds (fungi) can bloom on basement walls, in closets, in bathroom

POSSIBLE SOURCES OF HOUSEDUST PARTICLES

PLANT	ANIMAL	MANMADE
Mold spores	Pet dander	Acrilan
Cellulose:	Housedust mites	Dacron
cotton	Fragments:	Fiberglass
linen	feathers	Lycra
kapok	moths	Nylon
jute	cockroaches	Orlon
wood	spiders	Rayon
Pollen	silverfish	Spandex
	fleas	Paint
	mosquitoes	Plastic
	beetles	Rubber
	ants	Cigarette smoke
	Silk	Fireplace soot
	Felt	
	Furs	
	Horsehair	
	Wool	
	Mohair	
	Rabbit fur	
	Camel hair	

crevices, on wallpaper glue, on rotting vegetables. In hot, muggy climates it can even form on books, old shoes, and stacked magazines. As these molds mature, they send their spores floating throughout the house, to be breathed by the family living there. Conventional wisdom has it that the hay-fever season ends when ragweed is killed by that first November frost. Actually, ragweed ceases to be a problem a full month earlier. It's the *mold* that dies with the frost. The confusion arises because people allergic to ragweed pollen are often sensitive to mold as well.

Another common ingredient in housedust, surprising to most people, is a tiny arthropod called the housedust mite.[2] In one study a group of entomologists collected dust from sixty-four homes in the eastern half of the

United States, and they found a good quantity of house-dust mites in almost two-thirds of them.

The portion of housedust composed of plain dirt tracked in from outside isn't so worrisome, so far as health is concerned. But those other ingredients, the particles that come from *inside* the house, can affect a sensitive person in surprising ways. One patient came in not long ago with hives, and said that she had been suffering from them for years. Hives usually are a manifestation of a food allergy, but in this case I couldn't seem to locate the offending substance. So I decided to give her the full range of allergy tests—and to my surprise the only substance she reacted to significantly was housedust. That was on a Monday. I gave her an injection of housedust extract (to hyposensitize her), and another one that Friday. By the following Monday—one week after the first injection—the hives had cleared up completely. Since then her skin has stayed clear, and now she requires only an occasional maintenance injection. This is remarkable, because housedust rarely is associated with hives;

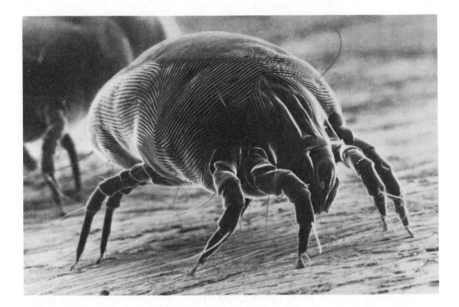

HOUSEDUST MITE is found in the housedust of most homes. Many people are more allergic to mites than to the other housedust components.

housedust allergy usually is manifested in rhinitis (inflammation of the nasal membranes) or such vague symptoms as the "winter blahs."

Housedust may be allergenic, but in itself it is rarely harmful; if you're not allergic, you can probably eat a cupful of the stuff without any more problems than a dry mouth and an unhappy stomach. But in some cases, particles wafting through the household air can be truly toxic. Not long ago I visited a neighbor who had just bought a wood-burning stove. To protect the wall, he was installing a sheet of asbestos, and he was using a saber saw to cut it to size. The dust swirled about his head, and every breath carried minute particles into his lungs. I was horrified. Here was an intelligent man who knew, from having read newspapers and magazines, of the deadly afflictions that workers in asbestos plants contract from breathing the dust. And here he was permitting this carcinogen in his own home. I was upset with my neighbor, and I was upset because the sheet had no cautionary label on it. Such material should have the same warning as iodine bottles, complete with skull and crossbones. Actually, sheet asbestos is *more* dangerous than iodine, because no adult is going to swallow iodine accidentally; yet my neighbor was breathing asbestos dust.

In fact, I'll go further: The federal government is charged with the responsibility of regulating substances that Americans ingest. The house, in a sense, is also an ingestant: It produces countless substances that find their way into our bloodstreams and our tissues. And to the body, the route of a chemical—whether through the stomach or lungs—matters not at all.

If full-disclosure labeling regarding the medical hazards of foods and drugs is required, then the government should also mandate health labeling on furnishings, clothing, household liquids, even building materials—because many of these, in the form of vapors or dust, are also taken internally.

As for my friend with the asbestos, I insisted that he shut off the saw and leave the room while I got a dust mask for him to wear. (Incidentally, the common masks sold by drugstores are virtually worthless for filtering out vapors and dust. You need the kind of mask found in large hardware stores, one that fits the face closely, and one into which you can screw various types of filtration canisters.)*

What happens when you breathe particles floating about in the air of your home? It depends on two factors: your particular degree of sensitivity and the makeup of those particles. One extreme example—and perhaps the most widespread source of indoor pollution—is tobacco smoke, which, among hundreds of different compounds, contains such harmful ones as carbon monoxide, nitrogen dioxide, hydrogen sulfide, hydrocyanic acid, and the highly active enzyme poison hydrogen cyanide. Long-term exposure to levels of hydrogen cyanide of about ten parts per million is considered dangerous; concentration in cigarette smoke is 1,600 ppm.

And the difference between doing the smoking yourself and rebreathing someone else's smoke is only a matter of degree. In fact, smoke from a cigarette burning in an ashtray contains almost twice the tar and nicotine of smoke inhaled from a cigarette, and so may be twice as toxic as smoke inhaled by the smoker.

The effect of tobacco smoke on the body is primarily as a toxin or series of chemical effectors, but in some cases it can act as an allergen too. One study of one hundred heavy smokers who had developed heart disease revealed that forty-four of them were actually *allergic* to the smoke.[3]

At any rate, most of the problems—at least most of the obvious ones—caused by household airborne particles can be traced to allergies. When people hear the word "allergy," most think either of food reactions in the form of skin problems and stomachaches, or of hay fever (which has nothing to do with hay and causes no fever) and its symptoms: the sneezing, the scratchy throat, the

* Suppliers of acceptable masks, as well as many other products discussed in this and succeeding chapters, can be found in Appendix C.

runny nose, the itchy, red, watery eyes. But these are only two of the many forms that allergy can have. Among the other most common:

Colic, painful intestinal cramps or bowel spasms affecting babies. It usually (but not always) is a reaction to cow's milk, but it can even be caused by mother's milk, if the mother has been drinking cow's milk. Typically, the baby's abdomen is hard and distended an hour or so after eating, and he cries piercingly, often for hours.

Infantile eczema, a skin rash of infants and children. Usually it is a reaction to milk or some other food, and it is likely to appear in children who have had colic. (Infants are most likely allergic to foods, while older children and adults are troubled additionally by airborne material.)

Respiratory allergy, manifesting itself in coldlike symptoms that settle mainly in the nasal membranes. This is the most common reaction of those sensitive to pollen—and it's called hay fever, or *pollinosis.* It often begins in childhood and continues throughout adulthood. The villain is not goldenrod or roses (there is no such thing as "rose fever"), but usually pollen from trees in springtime, grass during early summer, and ragweed in the fall. Dr. Frank L. Rosen of Maplewood, New Jersey, tells of a thirty-year-old woman who noticed a photo of a ragweed plant in his office. "Is this ragweed?" she asked. "It's growing very high outside my bedroom window. It even comes into the bedroom." Rosen comments that she was getting a pollen count of thousands when the reported count was only ten, and that when her husband cleaned out the backyard, her symptoms cleared up dramatically.[4]

Perennial allergic rhinitis, similar to simple pollinosis, but lasting all year. This is the "chronic catarrh" of our grandparents, and housedust (often coupled with mold or foods) is usually the villain.

Bronchial asthma, a recurring constriction or spasmodic contraction of the bronchi, or tiny air tubes of the lungs. The cells that manufacture mucus increase their output, the bronchial lining swells, the victim coughs and gasps for breath. Children suffer most, simply because their air passages are narrow to begin with. Nearly a quarter of all chronic school absenteeism can be traced to asthma.

Hives, itchy, pinkish bumps, something like mosquito bites without the puncture wound. Sometimes a reaction is so severe the spots blend into a single giant hive, and occasionally it progresses to the throat and vocal chords. Most hives are brought about by foods or medicines, but some people are allergic to heat or cold. Those sensitive to heat may develop eczema as a reaction to overheated rooms in winter, to warm-weather sunshine, even from exertion that raises the body temperature. Those who are sensitive to cold can induce hivelike swellings on the back of their hands simply by reaching into the refrigerator. The lips of one Denver boy I know of swell up whenever he eats ice cream, and one time, when he waded across an icy mountain stream, he threw up and nearly fainted. Some drownings, in fact, may have occurred when cold-sensitive individuals suffered whole-body reactions, leading to shock. The condition, relatively rare, is known as *cold urticaria*, and though its cause remains unknown, it is classified as an allergy because it has been successfully treated with antihistamines used to relieve conventional allergies.

Contact dermatitis, which often occurs with many cosmetics, is most familiar as poison ivy, poison oak, and poison sumac (to which at least half of all Americans are sensitive). Even if you stay indoors all the time, you aren't safe; if the family dog has been romping in a patch of poison ivy, you can pick it up from him. And you can get a good case simply by removing sap-coated shoes. Most virulent is the smoke from burning poison ivy or poison oak; it can affect skin, eyes, and even the throat and lungs.

These are some of the more common types of allergy. And their effects can be obvious or hidden, for the picture is even more complicated than it may seem.

For one thing, an allergy can manifest itself in unexpected ways. For another, one kind of allergy can evolve into a different kind. An asthmatic youngster can grow into an adult hay-fever victim (or the opposite), or someone who knows that he breaks out in a rash whenever he shakes the rug might suddenly find that he is no longer bothered with a rash, but now experiences extreme fatigue and depression; instead of a skin rash, he has developed mental problems. Few people continue through life allergic to only one thing; most develop other sensitivities, some keeping their old allergy, others dropping it. Some individuals respond to all allergens in the same way, while others may get hay fever from one, hives from another. And there's no way to know in advance who will get what allergies when, until the first attack occurs. A person usually develops allergies before his teens, yet I know one woman who showed no symptoms until she was in her mid-forties, when she suddenly found herself sneezing whenever she vacuumed.

Another fact that muddies the waters is that more than one substance might be necessary to cause a reaction—the primary allergen plus a "trigger." Someone sensitive to animal dander, for instance, might not show symptoms at all unless mold spore, a common trigger, is also present. One of my patients loves wine, and he drinks it with every evening meal—*except* when he eats with a friend who has a dog. Otherwise, he'd wheeze. He is mildly allergic to the mold in wine and to dog dander, but it takes both to trigger a reaction. Another patient complained that his food allergies were much worse after mid-September. What was happening, we determined, was that when the heating season started, his forced-air furnace began stirring up housedust, and the combination of his minor housedust allergy and his minor food allergy caused clinical symptoms. He could not tolerate foods he had eaten all summer.

The trigger doesn't even have to be physical. An asthma attack can be set off by emotional upset, even though the root cause remains organic.

Confusing things even more is the concept of *masked* allergy, first articulated by Herbert Rinkel, a Kansas City allergist who discovered the principle when he was trying to rid himself of his own allergic rhinitis. Masking is the *improvement* of symptoms when one submits himself to more of the same substance. Rinkel noticed that if when he was having an allergic reaction to a food (such reactions often last up to three days) he ate more of that food, he seemed to get *better*. Unfortunately, he eventually got worse (first relieved, then hungover) in sort of a hair-of-the-dog effect. As explained by Dr. Theron Randolph, noted Chicago allergist, this adaptation may be the only way such a person "knows to postpone or relieve his otherwise inevitable delayed hangover-like reactions, for only thereby does he remain 'normal' and without complaints. More commonly, however, such an adapted person simply eats what he likes and does what he is accustomed to do as often as desired without the slightest notion of 'adapting' or being involved in any addiction-type of response."[5] Adds Dr. Richard Mackarness, author of *Eating Dangerously:* "The mother who tells you that cow's milk used to make her child vomit soon after it was first introduced to the child's diet and boasts that, because she persisted with the milk feeding, her child can now take it and even likes it, is talking about masked food allergy."[6]

What the mother says is true, but she's harming the child in the long run, because the longer a person can avoid an allergen, the less susceptible he is to it. You're much more likely to develop an extensive reaction to poison ivy right after you get rid of a case of it than you will be two years later. And spend a year or two on a Tibetan mountaintop, and your hay fever will probably be much less bothersome when you return to the ragweed pollen of Ohio. At least until *next* year.

Still another confusion arises because a sensitivity might manifest itself in unsuspected ways. One morning not long ago a local clothing-store owner came to my office complaining of a severe rash on his hands. I explained to him that I could handle the problem in one of two ways: I could treat the symptom by prescribing an ointment that would relieve the itching and suppress the discoloration and eczema. He'd still be sick, I told him, but he wouldn't have to look at his illness. Or we could get to the bottom of it—spend the time to find out what was causing the reaction, then either eliminate the offender from his environment or treat specifically for the substance. In that case I wouldn't prescribe an ointment, because that would destroy my only *indicator system*.

"Let's do it right," he said. So we went through the standard procedures—extensive case history and sensitivity tests. He told me that his father got stomach cramps whenever he ate nuts, and that his grandmother used to sneeze all through the summer and once nearly died from a wasp sting. Those facts were significant; a tendency toward allergy is strongly hereditary. If both parents have allergies, the chances are at least two in three that a child will be allergic to something before the age of six, though not necessarily to the same thing as the parents.

I considered first the possible allergens that would be present both in the patient's clothing store and his home, because susceptible individuals are usually sensitized by those substances abundant in their environment. This is particularly true with allergies; in fact, you cannot be allergic to something with which you have had no contact. I know of a chemist in White Plains, New York, who gets all choked up whenever he works with guinea pigs, his chief laboratory animal. And if you're allergic to cats, chances are you're a cat lover, or at least live with one. That's why Europeans are allergic to neither poison ivy nor ragweed; those plants are not native to Europe. And that's why the first time someone is stung by a bee, there's no chance of an allergic reaction. (That venom, however, could prime his body for a severe reaction the *second* time he's stung.)

So I tested the clothing-store owner for substances found both in his business and home, found a number of common denominators, and suggested changing his environment to eliminate as many of them as possible. His clothing-store floor was being waxed once a week; he canceled the contract and stopped waxing his floors at home as well. He was using mothproofing substances in his store; I had him eliminate them from both his home and his business. He was also mildly allergic to wool and the accompanying dander; there wasn't much that could be done at the store, but he did install a filtering system in his home to cut down on the housedust, and he put his heavy wool living-room rug into storage, substituted synthetic blankets and pillows, and enclosed his mattress in a special dustproof cover.

In two or three weeks his hands had cleared up completely. On one of his last visits, he thanked me, then mentioned that his headaches had disappeared too. "What headaches?" I asked, because he had never mentioned them.

"I've had headaches all my life," he explained, "but I didn't think you'd be interested. I've been to headache clinics, consulted with a neurologist, tried a whole variety of medicines. I've spent a couple of thousand dollars trying to get rid of them, and finally decided that they are psychosomatic, and that I should see a psychiatrist." His headaches had been so frequent and so severe, he said, that he hadn't been able to go out on dates, and consequently he had remained a bachelor. Today, he still gets an occasional headache, but because he knows that the problem is environmental, he usually can pinpoint the cause. And he recently got married.

His headaches apparently were caused by some substance (or a combination of them) in his environment. Because of his reaction to skin tests, I strongly suspect that the primary troublemaking allergen was wool—something that he handled during the day, and, in the form of dust, breathed at night—aggravated by such other substances as mothball and wax fumes.

Wool is a common enough allergen, and a reaction to it shows the typical allergic mechanism at work. What happens is that the body's defense system mistakenly recognizes an allergen as an enemy, as a foreign substance, as something that must be eliminated. The immune system starts churning out a special kind of antibody to neutralize or annihilate the invaders, just as though they were disease germs. Now the body is "sensitized," primed for the next invasion. (If it doesn't come, the antibodies diminish in number; that's why the longer one can stay away from an offending substance, the better.) Now the allergen particles reappear. Whenever an antigen meets its specific antibody, they lock together like two magnets. One effect is that the small blood vessels dilate; another is that some of the specialized *mast* cells release histamine that circulates and settles all over the body, and those tissues that are particularly sensitive react, swelling and stimulating surrounding nerves, causing itching, burning, redness, and all the other uncomfortable symptoms associated with an allergic reaction. If the reacting organ is the skin, its blood vessels and cells—now swollen, distorted, broken down, and oozing their contents—appear as a rash. If it happens in the mucous lining of the nose, sinuses, or tracheobronchial tree, the glands produce surplus mucus, which the victim attempts to get rid of by coughing, sneezing, or nose blowing. (Some of the same general effects happen when the antibodies are doing legitimate battle with invading armies of a viral or bacterial infection. That's why allergic rhinitis can be so difficult to distinguish from an ordinary cold.) In the case of the clothing-store owner, the spillover from the battles not only caused the rash on his hands, but affected the blood vessels or tissues surrounding his brain. Result: headaches, tiredness, depression.

A few weeks after his last visit, the local newspaper printed a letter from him responding to a previously published article on headaches:

> I read with interest the article in your December 24 issue entitled, "Surprising Facts About Headaches," but as a headache sufferer I can tell you that there were no surprises in that column whatever. I know, as I have been suffering with headaches all my life, and the advice given is standard operating procedure. . . . When the "big men" complete their routine of head x-ray, EEG's and other tests, and everything checks negative, they say "you're experiencing tension headaches" and prescribe bigger and better

pills. This certainly is a tension filled world . . . but did you ever try to relax with the pain of a headache? It's not easy, especially when tension is not the cause.

The surprising fact is that not one of the countless doctors I visited in 48 years ever mentioned the word allergy as a possible cause of my pain. [Eventually I found out that] I was sensitive to the chemical world we have to live in. This is not to say that everyone is, but how many people are walking around "not feeling well" and not knowing why?

Spray your hair or underarm and inhale the chemicals; spray your sink and lavoratory and inhale the chemicals; leave that air-freshener open and inhale the chemicals; read the labels on the food packages on the supermarket shelves and ingest the chemicals. . . .[7]

The best defense against allergies, as in the case of this man, is avoidance. Either change the environment to weed out the offending substance, or change environments. Often an individual who is sensitive to substances around his home can determine for himself what the offenders are. (See procedures in Appendix A.) If not, he can consult an environmentally oriented physician to help in the detective work or to recommend medication.* That *something* be done about the airborne particles in your environment, in your home, is more important than you may realize.

The more energy you expend to fight off false armies of invading allergens, the less you have left, not only to attack *real* enemies of invading germs, but to do productive work at top efficiency. Allergies, to one extent or another, are debilitating. That accountant who was "coming down with something" all winter was simply too nonchalant to find out what was really wrong. As a result, his efficiency plummeted, his work suffered, and his income decreased. Eventually, he realized the fallacy of blundering through life in misery, and with help, he

* To find such a physician in your area, write to Robert Collier, M.D., Secretary, Society of Clinical Ecology, 4045 Wadsworth Blvd., Wheat Ridge, Colo. 80033.

tracked down the cause—that missing air filter from the furnace. After replacing the filter and moving his desk away from the airflow, he began to feel like his old self again—and to be productive.

Others are not so lucky. Those who push themselves no matter how terrible they feel (the hay-fever victim, for example, who insists on mowing his own lawn) are opening themselves possibly to more serious trouble, complications or even permanent damage. As a professional practitioner, I've spent years trying to cope with the effects of neglect: nasal polyps, chronic sinusitus, near loss of the sense of smell, diminished hearing, chronic fatigue, and a whole variety of emotional problems.

Poisonous Vapors That Surround You

About a year ago, in late spring, a patient came into the office for her regular injection for spring-grasses allergy. With her, for the first time, was her four-year-old daughter, Debbie. The child looked ill—sluggish and dull, with deep, puffy circles under her eyes. She seemed to be subnormal, with a striking lack of coordination, walking slowly and stiffly, almost like a marionette.

She had always been uncoordinated, sickly, and slow to learn, so her mother told me, and long ago her pediatrician had diagnosed her as "brain-damaged," apparently advising the mother to make the best of it.

But Debbie's condition was not a rarity in my office. I often see children exhibiting one or more of Debbie's symptoms. Usually it's simply a matter of intolerance to certain foods.

The fact that such intolerances can lead to a host of physical and emotional problems is well established. One outstanding researcher in this area is Ben F. Feingold, chief emeritus of the Kaiser-Permanente Allergy Foundation in San Francisco. Dr. Feingold's special interest is hyperactivity and learning disability in children. He has worked with hundreds of youngsters who are abnormally active, impulsive, and sometimes violent, and he estimates that there are nearly five million such children in the United States. Ordinarily such children are treated by powerful tranquilizers and amphetamines. But by carefully controlling his patients' diets, by removing foods with such ingredients as artificial coloring, synthetic preservatives, and salicylates, Feingold has eliminated wild behavior patterns in a large percentage of his patients.

It occurred to me that such sensitivity to foods or to the ingredients in foods might be causing the problems of four-year-old Debbie, so I suggested to her mother that we try a specialized elimination diet. Debbie would abstain from eating all but a very few classes of foods until an improvement was seen; then, one by one, specific foods would be added to the diet until a symptom again arose, and the responsible foods identified.

She agreed. But when there is one class of allergens active in causing problems, there often are others, so I considered alternative factors, using a detailed history questionnaire I had used over the past years. (It is duplicated, in part, in Appendix A.)

Did the family have pets? No. How often did members use perfume and aftershave? Rarely. Aerosols—deodorizers, hair spray, room fresheners—used a great deal? Hardly at all. Insecticides? Mothproofing? Antifungicides? No. What kind of kitchen stove? Natural gas. And *that* might be a clue. Are the problems seasonal? The mother thought for a few moments. Debbie always had problems, she said, but they seemed to be worse in the winter. I asked a final question: What kind of furnace did the house have? I had found in the past that gas is a major culprit. Perhaps the heating system was acting in concert with the stove in Debbie's home, producing fumes to which she was sensitive.

But her house had no furnace at all; it was heated electrically, and Debbie spent most of the time in her room. So much for that idea. I was about to move on to other points when Debbie's mother continued her sentence: ". . . and we use two kerosene space heaters to reduce the electric bill."

Space heaters, I knew, are a major pollution source in

an unhealthy house. Even heaters that are vented and well designed—and most are not—emit an amazing variety and quantity of vapors. And if a sensitive individual isn't yet directly affected by the fumes themselves, they may intensify reactions to other substances.

In this case, Debbie's mother had started using the auxiliary heaters about five years before. She bought them that September, in her second month of pregnancy, and during the next seven months had used one heater in the bedroom, the other in the kitchen. All the while, I suspected, the unborn baby was becoming sensitized. After the birth, Debbie's mother moved one heater to the nursery, where the baby breathed the fumes at night as she slept and during the day when she played. When she wasn't in her room, she was usually in the kitchen. Even during the warmer months, the child spent a considerable amount of time breathing fumes from the kitchen gas range. Sensitization, and subsequent trouble, was not surprising.

My main recommendations, of course, were two: Remove the space heaters from the house and disconnect the stove, substituting, for a few weeks, a hot plate. I further recommended that the mother remove as many synthetic chemicals as possible from Debbie's diet (food dyes, for example, and preservatives) and from her environment (floor waxes, cleaning agents and polishes), because such chemicals of petroleum origin often cross-react with fuel vapors. I advised no medication.

What Debbie was suffering from, I suspected, was petrochemical sensitivity, with its manifestation, in this case, *mental dysfunction,* a broad term that takes in a number of overlapping terms: hyperkinesis, neurological allergy, learning disability, and a variety of others. Such dysfunction can arise from numerous causes, such as inadequate diet of the mother or chemicals taken during pregnancy, inborn hormonal imbalances, injuries, genetic deficiencies—many things. But increasingly, researchers around the world are finding that a high percentage of mentally dysfunctioning children are suffering from some sort of sensitivity that has as its *target organ* the nervous system. In simple terms, the sensitizing entity is causing a "rash" of the brain. The same substance can affect different people differently, depending on which target organ is affected—in Debbie's case, the central nervous system. Some allergens—poison ivy and strawberries, for instance—affect the skin, and the result is dermatitis. Some work on the bronchial tract, leading to asthma. Some allergens act on the intestines, leading to diarrhea or spastic colon or gas or a "nervous stomach." And *mental dysfunction,* a great number of physicians now believe, is in many cases an assault on the brain by chemicals and foods that to the patient are intolerable.

Debbie's problem, I felt, would break down to a simple equation: A sensitive system plus stress equals mental dysfunction. The "sensitive system" is this particular child. Stress can be emotional (an argument with a friend), physical (a day too hot or too cold), or chemical (in Debbie's case, the petrochemical fumes).

A person reacting to a chemical attack often moves through a series of stages, perhaps recognizable, perhaps not. A familiar example is the alcoholic, whose physical source of stress is the alcohol. In the morning, because he was *deprived* of alcohol while asleep, he may be depressed. After a lunchtime drink or two, though, he feels relatively good. Then as the afternoon progresses with no drinks, he slides into depression again, only to move back into the normal, or even stimulated, range with the five-o'clock cocktail hour. That evening, however, he drinks too much, becomes overstimulated, then depressed again before he goes to sleep. And the next day it's much the same.

The alcoholic's response to his particular sensitizing agent is usually obvious. But a child sensitized to chocolate or soft drinks or cooking-gas fumes may respond to his chemical attack in unexpected or unrecognized ways. He may manifest such reactions as wheezing (asthma), stomachaches (irritated stomach lining), or chronic tiredness (brain dysfunction), leading to poor school grades. And of course he may also show such common reactions as stuffed nose, headaches, and rashes.[1]

Three weeks after the first visit of Debbie and her

mother, they returned, and I was amazed at the change in the child. She was smiling and happy. Those ugly circles had disappeared from beneath her eyes, and her skin had lost its sallowness. She was bright too—alert and interested in what was going on. And most dramatic of all, she was walking with only a hint of her former clumsiness.

I watched her throughout the year, watched her change from a subnormal child into a child physically normal and intellectually superior. During that time she did have one major relapse. It happened during a three-day Christmas visit to her grandparents' house. Her grandmother cooks on a gas range, and the house is heated by an old oil-burning furnace.

Debbie's growth into health was dramatic, but her problems with such vapors is by no means unique. Dr. Randolph and others involved in environmentally caused illnesses have run into many similar situations. One of Randolph's patients, a thirty-one-year-old housewife, "was first seen because of repeated bouts of rhinitis, fatigue, headache, myalgia, and low-grade temperature elevations suggestive of influenza," he reports. "She also complained of being dopey, groggy, unable to read comprehendingly or to think clearly. When these symptoms were intensified, she usually was depressed. At other times she was irritable, unsteady on her feet, and frequently dropped things."

During the summer his patient was somewhat better, particularly when she vacationed away from home. But when she returned, her symptoms surfaced again—which pretty much narrowed her problem to something in her house.

After a thorough study, Randolph recommended that she remove her gas range, gas refrigerator and gas water heater and that she substitute electrical equipment. When she complied, her condition improved by fifty percent, Randolph estimated. Nevertheless, she remained a sick woman. "When alternating depression and irritability-nervousness, dizziness and panic recurred," he wrote later, "the family decided to follow through with [my former] recommendation to replace the warm air furnace with hot water central heating, installing the furnace in the garage. The woman continued to improve. With the control of indoor air pollution, the avoidance of major chemically contaminated foods, and the adjustment of a few other areas, the patient has remained well." And with the mother's improved health, reported Randolph, "an unexpected development has occurred—the better health and behavior of the grade school children in this family; they are happier, less quarrelsome, and have greatly improved in their school work." [2]

The sources of the problems of Randolph's patient, Debbie, and untold thousands of others as well, are vapors—and the air of most homes is as polluted as a downtown city street during rush hour. One research team from Lawrence Berkeley Laboratory tested the air in six San Francisco Bay area homes selected as representative of "a cross section of typical American patterns of heating and cooking appliance use." They found the air in them not only containing such noxious vapors as carbon monoxide, nitric oxide and nitrogen dioxide, but in concentrations much higher than levels in the outdoor air, and up to four times the maximum recommended by federal guidelines. The researchers were appalled at their findings, and they were even more so when they speculated on the future. With America's increasing concern with energy conservation, homes in the 1980s will be built much tighter than they are now, further sealing in noxious vapors. "Older houses and most new houses have air exchange rates of one to two ACPH [air changes per hour]. Well-constructed new single-family houses have an air exchange on the order of only three-fourths to one per hour," they reported. "Energy conservation measures which would limit the air exchange rate in new houses to [only] ¼ to ½ ACPH are now being considered by state and federal governments." The researchers calculated that at the ¼-ACPH rate, carbon monoxide levels could rise to three times that of heavily polluted urban air, nitric oxide could jump to five times peak outdoor levels, and nitrogen dioxide could zoom to ten times the level of downtown areas.[3] One conclusion: Older houses may be more drafty, but in some respects, their inhabitants are probably better off. At least the air is fresher.

The difference between vapors and airborne particles is mainly one of size, but it also has some relationship to effect. Those who are bothered by particles in the air usually suffer from a conventional allergy. They may feel miserable, but airborne allergens in themselves don't kill. And at least in most instances, the victims know that something is wrong, and often they can track down the source themselves. They visit a friend with a cat and start wheezing; if they have any power of deduction at all, they know they're allergic to cats. With vapors, however, it may be a different story. Their effects are often more difficult to recognize, and are on the average potentially more dangerous than particles. One reason is that vapors penetrate the body's filtering system with ease— past the nose hairs, over the sticky bronchial substances, across the trachial cilia, right into the alveoli, the minute sacs deep in the lung where the exchange of carbon dioxide and oxygen in the blood takes place. Here they can pass easily through the permeable membranes and enter the bloodstream to be carried to all parts of the body.

Whereas particles are large clusters of molecules, vapors are single molecules floating through the air. In the home, vapors are usually a result of evaporation or combustion. A space heater produces fumes primarily as a result of the incomplete burning of fuels. But a second source of heater-produced vapors may be those airborne particles. The air that fuels the flame has suspended dust in it, and the dust, when burned (or even intensely heated), can break down into complex mixtures of gasses, often only remotely resembling the molecule clusters that were burned. So ordinarily innocuous particles from a synthetic rug, for instance, may be changed to virulent vapors simply because they've gone through the heating system.

Most of the year-round vapors in an average home (if nobody in the house smokes) comes about not through the heating system, but from evaporation. You slap some aftershave on your face and soon your family is breathing alcohol vapors. Coat kitchen cabinets with shellac, and the vapors produced as it dries—much more slowly than you think—float through the house for *weeks*. Some tiled-floor adhesives may take months to cease expelling vapors (especially with in-floor resistance heating). And it doesn't stop there. Many substances *continue* to "evaporate," even though they appear to have dried. Fiberglass insulation, for example, is often backed with kraft paper, the two layers cemented together with asphalt. Molecules of the substance slowly slough off, sublimating from the cement, then gradually disperse through the insulation and into the home. The amount is minute, but the evaporation is continuous, and over the years a person sensitive to petroleum derivatives may be inhaling the vapors, reacting, feeling listless or depressed or drugged. He has, in effect, encased himself in a cocoon of contamination of asphalt, augmented with continuously evaporating floor wax, with furniture polish, with disinfectant, with multitudinous other pollutants. Most of the problems with household vapors are much worse in the winter, when windows are closed and the sensitive individual is boxed in with the cause of his illness, breathing and rebreathing the vapors.

Most household vapors are insidious; you can't detect them. Many other harmful vapors, however, are readily discernible—and the sensor mechanism is the nose. The sense of smell is acute, 10,000 times more sensitive than the sense of taste, and your nose can give you more information than most people think possible.[4] One thing I've found through the years is that people who dislike certain odors often are sensitive to them. After all, the sense of smell (and of taste as well) is not something to give pleasure; it is a protective device. Sniff a piece of rotting meat and you're not very inclined to eat it. Take a drink and you automatically sniff it; champagne doesn't tickle the nose if the sipper holds his breath. A hundred thousand years ago the sense of smell was a principal means of survival.

The person who is most sensitive to certain fumes is

likely to be the first one to detect the smell when he walks into a room. I have no-smoking signs prominently displayed in the office, but sometimes a patient sneaks a cigarette anyway. My nurse is extremely sensitive to smoke (she becomes ill—nauseated and irritable), and when someone does light up in the outer office, even for a minute, she can detect it through two closely fitting doors. She knows when someone is smoking before anyone else in the office because she's more sensitive than any of the rest of us.

This response to odors is one of the areas I explore in my initial questioning of a new patient. I give him a list of common smells (scented soap, window-cleaning liquids, hair tonics and so forth) and ask whether he likes the smell, dislikes it, is neutral about it, or is sickened by it. Those patients who become ill in the presence of certain odors are, of course, sensitive to them. But I've found that often the person who simply *dislikes* particular smells is subsequently found to have been reacting physically to them.

Interestingly, many patients who state that they *like* certain odors also are adversely affected by them, particularly if exposed to the vapors regularly. Here again the adaptation syndrome is in effect; the individual has become used to inhaling the vapors, and even though he is reacting badly to them on a long-term basis, his immediate response is pleasure. The weekend mechanic who enjoys the smell of gasoline as he washes his lawnmower's carburetor may not realize that the exposure is the cause of his fuzzy thinking on Monday morning.

There is no conceivable way that the vapors from gasoline, incense, cologne, paint and other chemicals can benefit the body, although for most people short-term exposures may not be harmful. A general guide: *If you can't eat it, don't breathe it*—which rules out most of the odoriferous chemicals in the home. Nobody in his right mind would drink a room deodorizer, for instance, yet few hesitate to spray it around the house, breathing for the next few hours those same molecules of alien chemicals, which pass into the bloodstream even more easily than a sip of deodorizer. If a molecule of room deodorizer is in the bloodstream, what's the difference if it got there by way of the mouth, hypodermic needle, or lungs?

Incidentally, those so-called air fresheners that are supposed to deodorize, to rid the home of bathroom or kitchen smells, do no such thing. Odors are caused by the airborne dispersal of numerous molecules, and there is no known way of retrieving them, no chemical magnet. What the "deodorants" actually do is add *more* chemicals to the air, where they either mask the odor by overwhelming the nasal nerve endings with a stronger odor or temporarily poison the nerve endings so that they can't smell *anything* very well.

Such deodorizers may make the home superficially more pleasant, but they can have unpleasant, even disastrous, side effects. Here's an example:

About two years ago, in April, a worker in a local packaging company came to me complaining of numerous problems, among them (quoting from my original records), "lethargy, weakness, light-headedness, headaches, difficulty concentrating, decreased mental acuity, loss of visual acuity with difficulty in focusing, nausea, anorexia, increased intolerance to chemical odors." The man had been in good health until that January, with none of these symptoms.

After lengthy discussions and various tests, I found that his problem had originated in December, when his company became involved in packaging a concentrated room deodorant. During the process, some of the contents spilled, saturating the wooden floor. As a consequence, the man spent his working hours over the next five months breathing the vapors and developing a sensitivity. The problem that resulted was not, unfortunately, limited to a reaction to deodorant; the solution to that—avoidance—would be simple. The big trouble is this: As sensitivity develops to one chemical, it often spreads to related substances as well. So this packaging-company worker was now susceptible to chemicals of petroleum origin *as a group;* he was sensitive to such various household vapors as floor waxes and perfumes, as well as to artificial food dyes and the pesticide residue found in much of today's foods.

His prognosis at the time: poor, and it remains so today, two years later. His only hope is that over the long run he can avoid petrochemicals enough that his sensitization will diminish. But such avoidance is unlikely. The heavy exposure to a single petrochemical, an ordinary room deodorant, can trigger the classical symptoms of neurological allergy, and now the poor man must find some way to survive in a petrochemically polluted world.

This man had always disliked the smell of room deodorizers, and now his dislike is intense. But although the nose is highly sensitive, its usefulness is limited. You may be bothered by fresh varnish (encountered rarely and in heavy concentrations), but not even notice a leaking gas range or misadjusted heating system. Further, your nose may be fooled into thinking that the danger has passed. You walk into a room that has just been sprayed with an aerosol for "killing germs," for instance, and it smells terrible. Ten minutes later, though, you don't notice it; the odor has gone. Actually, it hasn't. You've simply gotten used to it. Your nasal nerve endings have done their job—warned you of a *change* in the environment—and now they ignore the smell and set themselves to detect something else.

The materials around the house that can produce noxious fumes can be counted by the dozens. Some are obviously toxic, others less so. Here is a breakdown of the home substances I've found to be most troublesome:

Fuels

These top the list. Kerosene and utility gas, both natural and artificial (in ranges, furnaces, refrigerators, or clothes driers) is perhaps second only to cigarette smoke as the worst home pollutant, hazardous to the susceptible both through pipe-joint leaks (*most* systems leak at least a little) and in the burning process. Every pilot light adds its own fumes. Says Dr. Randolph, who has caused more than 500 gas-fired kitchen ranges to be removed from his patients' homes: "Air contamination arising from gas kitchen ranges cannot be adequately eliminated by such partway measures as increasing ventilation in the kitchen, keeping the kitchen door closed, installing a kitchen exhaust fan, turning off the stove's pilots, disconnecting the stove but leaving it in the room, or even by turning off the gas at the point where the gas line enters the house."[5] His solution is to remove from the house either all gas lines or the patient.

Oil tanks in the basement often seep, contaminating basement air and eventually the whole house. A floor once flooded with oil can give off vapors for years.

Fireplaces add considerable pollutants, puffing smoke and vapors into living rooms when the wind shifts. In some conditions, smoke coming out of the furnace chimney has been blown *down* an adjacent fireplace chimney.

And kerosene space heaters are such a menace they should be legally banned.

Paint and Varnish Removers

All liquid and paste paint removers are suspect, and most are downright terrible. One active substance in many products is benzene, a substance contained also in cleaning agents and rubber cement (such as used for tire patches). In 1977, researchers from the National Institute for Occupational Safety and Health bought a standard paint remover containing 52 percent benzene from a local department store, and in an ordinary two-car garage stripped the paint from an end table while measuring the fumes. They found that a person exposed for five minutes would inhale more than forty-three times the amount permitted by federal occupational exposure standards. Concluded the researchers: "Until regulatory action is taken by appropriate government agencies, or voluntary action is taken by responsible industries, concerned citizens [must] take action to protect themselves."[6] Since 1928, exposure to benzene has been linked with leukemia, yet it remains widely used in the home. The Consumer Product Safety Commission is currently considering a ban on benzene-containing products for home use.[7]

Most paint removers containing ingredients other than benzene are almost as bad. Dr. Richard D. Steward, of the Department of Environmental Medicine, Medical College of Wisconsin, tells of a retired executive who decided to strip a wooden chest of drawers. He applied a paint and varnish remover containing the common ingredient methylene chloride, worked on the chest for three hours in his basement, relaxed for an hour, then suffered a heart attack.

He survived. Two weeks after discharge from the hospital, he decided to complete his paint-removing job. After three hours of stripping, he again suffered a heart attack and was rushed to the hospital. Again, he lived.

This time it was six months before he felt well enough to return to his paint-removing chore. With the help of his wife, he worked slowly for two hours. Two hours after that, his chest began to pain. He collapsed. This time he didn't make it to the hospital.[8] Conclusion: If you *must* use paint remover, do the job outside, stand upwind, and use a charcoal filter mask and protective gloves.

Paints and Varnishes

Like paint removers, paints and varnishes can themselves cause major problems as they evaporate. I've noticed over the years a direct relationship between freshly painted rooms and an exacerbation of whatever happens to be wrong with my patients—eczema, hay fever, arthritis, depression, whatever. Any kind of paint should be used only with the windows wide open and a fan blowing out the air. The sensitive person should time his vacation so that he is away as the paint is drying. And if he moves into a freshly painted apartment, he should try to overlap the time between residing in the old and the new domicile by at least two weeks, so he won't be boxed in with the fumes. The *best* advice is not to use paint at all. If you must, paint in the spring, and leave the windows open all summer. Some sensitive individuals will detect paint fumes for three months or more after application.

Alcohol from evaporating shellac and brush-cleaning solvents also may cause reactions. Rubbing alcohol can cause acute reactions in a chemically sensitive person—a point that should be made to the administration at the hospital admission desk.

Polishes

All polishes—from shoe to furniture to silverware polish—should be used outdoors or with the windows wide open, or better, be avoided entirely. One of my patients once complained of moderate tiredness and some loss of concentration, then passed it off with, "Oh well, I guess these things happen as you get older." They don't, at least not in this case. Her problem was traced to frequent use of a petroleum-based furniture polish.

Medicine Cabinets

Medicine cabinets often contain more medical problems than solutions, harboring such volatile substances as tincture of iodine and tincture of Merthiolate, nail polish and its remover (acetone), and a hundred other substances that slowly evaporate, bathing the bathroom in a chemical fog. My advice: Eliminate everything you can do without—an action that probably will nearly empty the cabinet. Or keep everything that's volatile in a cabinet in the garage.

Insecticides

A substance whose only purpose is to kill by poisoning should be treated with utmost caution, should be used only in emergencies, and of course should not be taken into the system. That's only logical. And yet half of the population seems to be intent on committing slow-motion suicide. One by one, high-powered biocides are being federally banned and removed from the marketplace, and anyone who is at all aware knows that any pesticide is potentially lethal. (The cellular metabolisms of insects and man have more similarities than differences.) And yet the home insecticide market remains a multimillion-dollar industry. Not only are sprays used throughout most American homes, but some people even hang poison-saturate strips in the nursery, forcing babies to breathe the slowly evaporating vapors, with God only knows what long-range consequences.

The harmful effects of insecticides are so well documented that a review here would seem to be superfluous. Here are a few items, however, that you may not know:

• Some insecticides, once applied, can never really be removed. The only thing to do with a heavily fumigated house is to move.

• Many insecticides are relatively insoluble in water, and are instead dispensed in petroleum-based solvents, to which a large number of individuals are sensitive. So not only are the principal ingredients a potential source of trouble, but the vehicle is too.

• Some rugs are treated with insect toxins as part of the manufacturing process. They can't be easily removed by cleaning, and even if they could be, it wouldn't matter; many professional cleaning establishments routinely use mothproofing substances when they treat rugs and blankets. And so a health-aware homeowner should specify that he wants no special "service," just the cleaning.

• A particularly surreptitious source of trouble are insect repellents, insecticides, or fungicides in wallpaper paste. If large areas of your home are wallpapered, you may be living in an insecticide-and-fungicide-lined box.

Other Potential Problem Areas

PLASTICS: These are an unsuspected font of misery for the chemically susceptible. The big offenders here are *soft* plastics—handbags, shower curtains, upholstered materials, and pillow and mattress cases, for example. Such hard plastics as Formica countertops, vinyl floors, and Bakelite products rarely cause problems, although cases of individuals sensitive to the plastic of a telephone have been reported.[9] (Others are affected by cotton wads impregnated with mold inhibitors found in many telephone mouthpieces.) Except for clothing, the more flexible a plastic, and the more odor it has, the more likely it is to produce troublesome vapors.

RUBBER: Some housedust-allergic patients have substituted sponge-rubber pillows and mattresses to guard against exposure, only to find the vapors from the rubber even more annoying than the bedclothes dust. Other household rubber sources include rubber rug pads and rug backing, upholstery, seat cushions, typewriter pads, rubber-tiled floors, and electrical insulation of electric blankets.

HOME OFFICE SUPPLIES: If a person develops symptoms while working in his study, he might suspect vapors from marking pencils, certain carbon papers, and some typewriter ribbons. Evaporating oil from the typewriter may also be to blame (as may oil from motors of other home equipment, or from air conditioners using oil-impregnated fiberglass filters).* Particularly troublesome to some people is the odor of fresh newsprint. Solution: Place the newspaper in the oven for a few minutes (to dry the ink) or read it later in the day.

REFRIGERANT GAS: Refrigerators, deep freezes, and air conditioners may leak, causing symptoms among the susceptible. Such gas (fluorocarbon) is the same that is being eased out as a propellant of pressurized cans of hair sprays, whipped toppings, drugs, and other substances.

CONIFER PRODUCTS: Hardwood and its products are not usually cause for concern, but if one becomes sensitized to evaporating lacquer, varnish, or paint that con-

---

* If you *must* oil a machine, use medical-grade mineral oil, obtainable from a pharmacy. This too may cause problems, but it's the best I've found.

tains turpentine—all of them wood products—he may also develop sensitivity to vapors produced from slowly drying softwood paneling (pine, spruce, and other conifers), which may take years to evaporate their resins. He may also be sensitized to burning fireplace wood, cedar closets, Christmas trees, and to such pine-scented items as floor cleaners and other cleaning agents, household deodorizers, bath oils, and shampoos.

Some chemically sensitive people have been breathing household vapors that are to them toxic for so long they no longer know what's it like to feel well. Only when the source of their problem has been removed do they begin to realize the real joy of living in a healthy environment, and in a healthy body.

Electrical Charges in the Air

Every so often in Austria, a steady, warm, dry wind comes blowing down from the ridges of the Alps. It is called the *foehn*, and it is evil. It causes noses and eyes to itch, stomachs to complain, minds to muddle. It brings with it general malaise and tension, diminished sex drive, and depression. Marriage problems intensify, automobile accidents increase, suicides rise, and crime rates soar by as much as 20 percent. When it passes, things abruptly, miraculously, return to normal. It is a wind, the Austrians say, that can drive men mad.

Robert H. Moser, former editor of the *Journal of the American Medical Association,* tells of how he learned of the foehn when he first began practicing in Salzburg:

"One day I admitted a young soldier who had suffered a brain hemorrhage from a ruptured berry aneurysm [a balloonlike swelling of any artery]." Moser consulted with a neurosurgeon friend, who agreed that an operation was imperative. "I recall his words most vividly: 'Yes, it will not be difficult. . . . We will do it in a few days, after the foehn stops blowing.' I turned and stared at him in astonishment; what a curious, superstitious statement from this sophisticated, internationally trained surgeon. He smiled: 'Don't be so amazed. After all, there is no rush about it, and after you've been in

Austria awhile you will understand. When the foehn blows—things just go wrong. Wounds become infected, sutures break, nasty little complications arise. Nurses fret and cry easily. A surgeon's hands are not as sure. I don't know why it happens, but it does. I defer all elective surgery until the foehn stops blowing. We'll wait.' "

And so they waited. And over the years, Moser learned that the surgeon's words were more than folklore or superstition.[1]

Such a phenomenon, such an "evil wind," is not peculiar to Austria. Twice a year the dusty *sharav* sweeps across Africa and the Sinai Peninsula, carrying with it general distress. The hot, arid, hazy *sirocco* blows a sense of oppression over Sicily and southern Italy, and in Syria, a similar wind is called *simoon*, which means "poisoning." Across the northwestern Mediterranean coastal plains it is the *mistral*, the "witches' wind," and it, too, brings general unease, nervousness, headache, and a multitude of other ills. Greece has its *meltemia*, the ill wind that Homer called *etesiae*. And in North America, the Santa Ana wind brings a touch of madness to Californians, the winter *Chinook* carries misery to residents of parts of the Rockies, and the summer winds of the Arizona-Mexican desert brush the ranchers with what the Indians call "wind sickness."

What are these winds, and what strange substance in them causes such widespread unhappiness? Scientists now know that the mysterious ingredient is electricity—positively charged particles that ride on the air currents, particles that somehow influence our cells, which in themselves contain, and are governed by, tiny electric charges. Among other things, ions seem to influence moods and to explain why rheumatic joints act up before rain, why some animals grow skittish, and why ants block their entrances before storms.

Nature produces ions by a variety of means: by cosmic rays and the action of sunlight, by wind and weather fronts, by radioactive elements in the soil. Other factors include barometric pressure, temperature, humidity, the proximity of large bodies of water, the nature of surrounding surfaces, and the elevation. Even air pollution has an effect; the number of ions decreases as the pollution rises.[2] The normal ratio at sea level is about five positive to four negative ions, with a total count over land averaging somewhere between 1,000 and 2,000 ions per cubic centimeter. Man can generate ions with radio-isotopes, high-energy radiation, and charged wires or coils. Ion concentration is usually higher in summer than winter, higher when the temperature is elevated, higher during the day than at night, higher when the weather is clear rather than cloudy, and even higher when the moon is full. (Interestingly, this may partially explain why the full moon seems to have such an influence on living things. For example, when two researchers from the University of Miami School of Medicine ran fifteen years of Dade County homicides through a computer, they found a significant relationship between the homicide rate and phases of the moon.[3])

In the mountains (traditional location of European sanitariums), the concentration becomes much higher. And in all these situations, the human being has more energy, is more optimistic, and simply feels better.

Technically, an ion is an atom that has either lost an electron or has gained an extra one. All atoms have a basic structure similar to a bull's-eye target. The center is the nucleus; the outside rings are electrons and their pathways, with the electrons spinning around like merry-go-round horses. The central nucleus has a positive charge, while peripheral electrons have a negative charge. Ordinarily, they balance each other; the atom as a whole is neutrally charged. But if for some reason it gains an extra electron, it becomes negatively charged, and if it loses one, it becomes positive. In those cases it's called either a negatively or positively charged ion. If it clumps together with other particles, it becomes an ionized molecule.

What has all this to do with a healthy house? Two things: (1) Researchers now believe that ions in the air have a profound effect on human beings, and (2) a householder, by deciding where he lives, of what materials his house is constructed, and what furnishing he uses, can do something about it.

Exactly how ions affect people is still somewhat obscure. But *what* they do to the human being is now becoming clear. One researcher, Professor Felix Gad Sulman, head of Hebrew University's Department of Applied Pharmacology in Jerusalem, found that ions affect brain waves. Volunteers subjected to heavy concentrations of negative ions show, through EEG readings, that alpha rhythms tend to move to the forward part of the brain. Other authorities have found that negative ions stimulate human cilia—those tiny, hairlike organs that line the lower throat—while positive ions depress them; and negative ions speed delivery of oxygen to tissues, while positive ions slow down the delivery.

What is looked upon as perhaps the most significant finding in recent years is the discovery that ions apparently affect the release of serotonin, a high-powered and many-faceted mediator that participates in such varied processes as blood-pressure regulation, inflammation control, the transmission of nerve impulses, and moods.

It may even be the stabilizer that keeps us sane—at least that is the possibility suggested by British physiologist J. H. Gaddum during studies of the hallucinogen LSD (lysergic acid diethylamide), a structural cousin of serotonin that can induce schizophreniclike states. Further studies at the Rockefeller Institute of Medical Research suggested that certain forms of mental disease may be due to disturbances in the metabolism of serotonin.

The discovery of the ion/serotonin relationship was made by Dr. Albert Krueger, emeritus professor of bacteriology at the University of California, Berkeley, probably the best-known researcher in the ion-and-health field. He experimented for three years with mice, raising them in air with various degrees of positive and negative ion levels. He then wrote in the *Journal of General Physiology* that excessive positive ions, such as found in foehn winds, apparently trigger an overproduction of serotonin, and that the immediate effect is hyperactivity, followed by gross tiredness, and eventually anxiety and probably depression as well.[4]

Hebrew University's Professor Sulman, during a subsequent four-year study of serotonin, also made a fascinating discovery. Serotonin, it had been known, is occasionally found in the urine of human beings, but only when they are undergoing anxiety or emotional stress. When Sulman tested 200 men and women who complained of the Israeli sharav wind, he found that their bodies produced an average of ten times as much serotonin as during the windless season. The meaning? Fred Soyka, author of *The Ion Effect,* speculates that "it seems likely that while adrenaline is produced in response to threats of survival that we can detect with one of our five senses, serotonin is our body's response to threats that we can't perceive through our senses."[5] Such as electrical stress.

Although Sulman believes that everyone is adversely affected by heavy concentrations of positive ions, "weather-sensitive" people—making up about one-quarter of the population—are, in effect, poisoned by their own excessive serotonin when positive ions cause the mediator to be released into the system. The results are various: headache, insomnia, chest pains, breathing problems, and a whole raft of emotional troubles. Sulman also found that excess positive ions over the years rob the body of its ability to withstand stress, leading to metabolic exhaustion. And finally, he learned that positive-ion poisoning interferes with the workings of the thyroid, which, among a number of other functions, helps regulate the production of histamine. Those who live in the path of the sharav wind, Sulman discovered, suffer from an excess of histamine, and that fact (at least in part) accounts for complaints of watery eyes, itching noses, and asthmalike breathing problems.[6]

Using his discoveries, with ten years of research behind him, Sulman then attempted to duplicate some of Dr. Krueger's work, using, instead of rats, human beings. When he allowed victims overcharged by the wind to breathe air laden with artificially produced negative ions, fully three-quarters of them were relieved. (Why *everyone* wasn't helped remains unknown.) He also found that sufferers of the wind could be helped by drugs that prevent serotonin buildup.

Other researchers found that ions seem to have different effects on various ages. The positively ionized *khamsin* provides a good example. Young people in its path tend to develop headaches and nausea. They are irritable, tense, and occasionally violent. Older people, on the other hand, tire more easily than usual, becoming depressed and lethargic. And sometimes they have near blackouts.

Negative ions have just the opposite effect: energy, well-being, glee, especially in the young. Dr. D. W. Hansell, an RCA Laboratories research fellow and an authority on ions, tells about the time he noticed a negative-ion influence on his ten-year-old daughter: "We were outside watching the approach of a thunderstorm. . . . I knew that clouds of negative ions were filling the air. Suddenly my daughter began to dance across the grass. There was a radiant look upon her face. She leaped upon a low boulder, threw her arms wide to the dark sky, and cried, 'Oh —I feel wonderful!' "[7]

What had happened was this: The clouds and the weather front brought with them a superabundance of positive ions that moved in well before the storm. (Ions often arrive hours or even days ahead of time, which explains why arthritis and old wounds hurt before storms.) Eventually, still miles away from the child, the charges grew so large that lightning discharged. But when the storm arrived, it brought with it negative ions, with that typical smell of fresh, new-mown hay (which, incidentally, can be duplicated in the laboratory simply by generating negative ions). The atmosphere flipped from positive to negative, from one of heaviness and depression to a glorious skyful of negative ions that made the air seem fresh, clean, invigorating, and filled the child with joy.

I've noticed similar marked changes, both short- and long-term, in my own patients. One, for example, is a young inventor who, when he lived in lower New York State, complained that he didn't have the energy he felt he should have, and that he was sleepy most of the time. In addition, he was generally depressed, and much of the time a little angry as well. Eventually he moved to California, to a cabin high on a mountain. Recently he telephoned me to let me know how well he was doing: "Remember that I used to sleep ten hours a night, and took naps every afternoon too? Now I need only six hours sleep, and I feel much more energetic than when I was sleeping ten. That's four extra hours a day. I figured out that if I live another forty years, I'll add the equivalent of nearly seven years to my life—productive years." And he'll live not only longer, but better.

The factor, I believe, is *where* he lives—not only far from megalopolitan pollution, but in an electrically superior environment. In fact, I feel that human beings know at some intuitive level where to go for such an environment. For vacations we head to an electrically benevolent environment—to the seashore or to the mountains, not to Times Square. You come back refreshed and think it's simply because you've been away from work, and actually that might have a lot to do with it. But so does that time spent in electrically compatible surroundings. The spas of Europe owe much of their success to their locations—in areas rich in radioactive soils, often near natural and artificial waterfalls; the air in many such places contains a thick concentration of ionized air, with a high ratio of negative to positive ions. When measurements were taken at a Russian spa near a waterfall, scientists were amazed to find 100,000 ions per cubic centimeter, while just a half-mile away the count was a normal 1,500.

At the oceanside, the combination of spray and sea breezes rubbing against the waves produces high concentrations of negative ions. You find the same thing even in the home shower, which is one reason why a shower is so invigorating, so refreshing.[8]

Sometimes just a few miles makes the difference. The Hudson Valley, where my practice is located, has its own miniature foehn. At least that's my theory, resulting from sixteen years of clinical observation. Some patients, beset by numerous respiratory and other ills, find great relief simply by taking a brief ride fifty or sixty miles west, to the western slope of the Catskills, only one or two thousand feet higher than their homes. One of my patients who has eczematous skin rash (she is allergic to a variety of foods) lives in Kingston, New York. Occasionally she spends a few days with her father, in Roxbury, high in the Catskills. There, her symptoms abruptly disappear, and she can eat anything she desires. But when she returns, so does her eczema, and she must go back to her strict diet. A number of factors could account for the effects—change of pollen species, varying levels of mold, industrial pollution, psychosomatic effects—but I believe the principal cause to be the electrically beneficial air of the higher elevations. In fact, some researchers have found that the incidence of heart attacks is less at higher elevations.[9] And even this, I believe, is the result of ionically superior air.

Even if one lives in an ionically ideal area, however, the effects are often negated by modern houses, offices, and apartments, in which technological man seems to have created his own built-in foehn—a *reverse* pollution, in which beneficial entities are removed. In 1969, the Polish researcher B. Maczynski ran a two-week study of a typical office containing four workers. As each day wore on the ion concentration fell to an average of only thirty-four positive and twenty negative ions per cubic centimeter.[10] In another study, this one run in a light-industry area of San Francisco, the active ion count in most indoor locations was twenty to thirty-five per cubic centimeter.[11] These concentrations compare with an average count of more than a thousand ions per cubic centimeter in the open countryside. The implications are startling: The tiredness and tension one feels after a hard day at the office may be caused more by the seven hours in an ion-depleted atmosphere than by the actual workload.

One reason for ion depletion indoors is that negative

ions tend to attach themselves to particles of dust and pollution and lose their charge, or cluster together to become large ions, which apparently have little effect on the body.[12] Another reason is that they attach themselves to metal fans, filters, and ducts in central air-conditioning systems and are subsequently lost. According to RCA's Dr. Hansell, "high-velocity air-distributing systems in some of the most modern skyscrapers are believed to be particularly bad in this respect. This explains why so many people in them feel depressed, and have an urge to throw open a window." And that goes for central air-conditioning systems in the home as well.

Hansell also points out that our distant ancestors, over a million years of evolutionary development, "lived, literally, with their feet on the ground, and so were electrically grounded." In contrast, he says, we are electrically insulated from ground much of the time, and so we are creating a situation in which charges can be stored on ourselves. "Often our bodies are at potentials far different from ground and our surroundings. These potentials can have large effects upon the ratio of positive to negative ions we absorb from the air and upon their total number."

That means that if a person's body somehow becomes negatively charged, it will attract positive ions like iron tacks to a magnet. How could that happen? Easy, in the modern home. All you have to do is walk across a new wool carpet with rubber- or leather-soled shoes in winter and you'll become highly charged, so much so that when you touch another person the charge jumps the gap with a spark. If your charge happens to be negative, which is likely, then positive ions in the air will constantly be flocking to you. (*Like* charges repel; opposites attract.)

"It would be better," says RCA's Hansell, "if we could put the leather or rubber on the floor and wool on our feet," adding that "the time may come when clothing and room surface materials will be graded and labeled according to their positions in the triboelectric series," a classification of materials by their ability to generate electricity by friction.[13] And I believe that future weather forecasts will include not only temperature, pressure, and humidity, but ion concentration.

Dr. Krueger, the bacteriologist from the University of California, foresees the day when people will regulate the ion count in their homes "just as we now have set limits for temperature, relative humidity, air turnover, etc. The goal then will be to maintain air-ion concentrations and ratios at levels approximating those existing in nature."[14] Adds Fred Soyka:

> We will also almost certainly reach the point where all building materials will be approved only if they are not likely to upset the ion effect. And I expect that all furnishings and clothing made with synthetic fibers will have either their positive or negative potential listed along with the washing and cleaning instructions. Better still, there may be legislation demanding that these synthetics be treated chemically to neutralize their electrostatic potential entirely.[15]

Meanwhile, householders can select furnishings and materials for optimum ion control (as outlined in Chapter 6) and watch the weather. When the temperature is rising and the barometer falling, the probabilities are that the air will be swarming with positive ions. As science writer Robert O'Brien puts it, "We should then brace ourselves for quarrels at the breakfast table, for perversity in our children, for short tempers at the office. If possible, we should avoid matters which hinge upon the cooperation or agreement of others."[16]

In other words, wait for those crystal-clear days of rising pressure and falling temperatures. Or move to the mountains.

The Electromagnetic Waves in Your Home

In December 1971 the Electromagnetic Radiation Management Advisory Council, a nine-member group appointed by the White House, issued a little-publicized report to the American people: "Program for Control of Electromagnetic Pollution of the Environment." Among its major findings:

• "The electromagnetic radiations emanating from radar, television, communications systems, microwave ovens, industrial heat-treatment systems, medical diathermy units, and many other sources permeate the modern environment."

• "This type of manmade radiation exposure has no counterpart in man's evolutionary background; it was relatively negligible prior to World War II."

• "Power levels in and around American cities, airports . . . industry and homes may already be biologically significant."

• "Unless adequate monitoring and control, based on a fundamental understanding of biological effects, are instituted in the near future, in the decades ahead, man may enter an era of energy pollution of the environment comparable to the chemical pollution of today."

• "Research in the field of long-term, low-level effects of electromagnetic radiation on living systems has been near a standstill in this country. . . . The consequences of undervaluing or misjudging the biological effects of long-term, low-level exposure could become a critical problem for the public health."

In essence, what the report was saying is this: Americans are surrounded by all manner of man-made electromagnetic radiation—radiant energy in the form of waves moving through space—never before experienced by any species, and the long-term consequences are unknown and might be enormous, perhaps disastrous. The question constitutes one of the most complicated, baffling, and controversial medical problems ever confronted.

To get a grasp on the possibilities, a little background:

Every living thing is continually bathed in an electrical climate, indoors and out, in the desert and in the city. In addition to the particles or ions covered in Chapter 4, the electrical climate includes electromagnetic waves. Scientists studying such waves customarily arrange them according to length and frequency. At one end are the long, low-frequency radio waves, which may stretch for thousands of miles and vibrate as slowly as ten cycles a second (or ten *hertz*, or *Hz*). At the other end are the gamma rays, incredibly short (measured in angstrom units, or ten-millionths of a millimeter), vibrating at such high frequencies that the figures are almost meaningless: millions of trillions of Hz. Between them, in descending order of frequency, are X-rays, ultraviolet radiation, visible light, infrared (or heat) radiation, and microwaves. If a person's eyes were sensitive to all these wavelengths, then he would know no night, no darkness, even with his eyes closed; the entire sky would glow, the earth bathed in an ocean of waves, in so much "light" that sight, as we know it, would be meaningless.

In addition, other kinds of waves or "influences" are present that ordinarily are not placed within the confines of the electromagnetic spectrum: gravity, for example, and the earth's magnetic field, which has been shown to be subject to slow pulses, and little-understood phenomena brought about by solar flares and giant magnetic storms raging on the sun, hurling solar-wind atomic particles into space and onto earth.

Many body functions—hormone levels, temperature, serum iron levels and alertness, for example—vary throughout the day in regular cycles. The timing mechanism for the clock remains a mystery; it seems *not* to be internal, nor something cued by light, barometric pressure, or temperature. It's something else, probably something in the electromagnetic environment.[1]

Some of the waves that human beings are bathed in are natural; others are man-made. Most natural electromagnetic phenomena originate in the sun, and the bulk of these are obvious. Man can see (by visible light), he gets sunburned (from ultraviolet rays), he feels heat (from the infrared). Other natural waves are not so apparent. Some come from far off in the galaxy—X-rays, for instance, and gamma rays.

The ancient environment, the subtle rhythms of the universe, has been with *Homo sapiens* since the beginning. He's been surrounded by natural electromagnetic fields that until recently have remained relatively constant. Man himself is an electrical organism. The communication within and between all the cells of his body is a function of electrical charges. (An electrocardiogram records the total electrical pulses of all the individual muscle cells generated by the action of the heart.)

The surface of the body is surrounded by a charge and its associated electrical field. Dr. Robert O. Becker, an orthopedic surgeon at Syracuse Veterans Administration Hospital and New York's Upstate Medical Center, along with a colleague, physicist Charles Bachman, has mapped this electrical field, using sensitive electrodes. They found that it is generally negative at the forehead, positive behind the brain and along the larger nerve groups of the upper shoulders and lower back, and largely negative at the arms and legs. The polarity, they discovered, can be influenced by outside forces. Said Becker in testimony given before the State of New York Public Service Commission:

We predicted that external electromagnetic fields should produce physiological and functional changes in living organisms. . . . The result of these experiments [of fifteen years' duration] have conclusively indicated that such fields *do* have an effect upon living organisms.[2]

For example, when a person is given a general anesthetic, says Becker, the reading at the forehead gradually shifts from negative to zero. Another example he cites is that of the regeneration process. When a salamander's leg is cut off, the limb's electrical charge switches abruptly from negative to positive, then gradually shifts back to its normal negativity as the leg regenerates. When Becker surrounds the growing limb with an artificial, negative current charge, the regeneration process speeds up.

He went one step farther and attempted to achieve limb generation in mammals. When he applied a negative charge to the severed limbs of rats, total regeneration did not occur, but it *began;* both bones and tissues showed the beginnings of regrowth.[3]

Viewing the results of this and other experiments, Becker hypothesized that more subtle electromagnetic fields might also influence organisms. So on a hunch he correlated solar activity with admissions to six New York State psychiatric institutions and found that the highest admission rate occurred during times of massive solar storms, then diminished again as the magnetic intensity lowered.[4]

"The response to our reports [that electromagnetic forces might have effects upon living organisms]," says Becker, "has changed from rejection just over a decade ago through amused disbelief to—at present—enthusiastic acceptance."[5] Changes in geomagnetic fields might explain a series of medical mysteries, Becker believes— such things as the reason why ulcers are more likely to flare up in the spring and fall, and why susceptibility to infection seems to vary with the seasons.[6]

Such natural electromagnetic, gravitational, and subtle cosmic forces of the ancient environment not only have an effect on living things, but, scientists are finding, seem to be *essential* to life. If you place living entities—bacteria, plants, animals—in what are called

Faraday cages, in environments that block out virtually all of the background radiation, strange things happen to them, most of them bad.[7] Bacteria change in size and shape, and usually reproduce more slowly. Termites lose their sense of direction. Flies reproduce more slowly for about seven generations, then, in what seems to be an effort to make up for lost time, reproduce at a *higher* rate than usual. And plants in Faraday cages usually grow weak and spindly.[8]

In an experiment directed by NASA, mice were kept in cages designed to eliminate as many waves of the natural electromagnetic spectrum as possible. A review of the experiment stated:

Initially . . . the females bore fairly large and quite normal progeny. By the fourth generation reproduction ceased. But even earlier, in the second generation, there were more miscarriages and cannibalism than [in a control group]. A large number of the mice kept in shielded conditions became inactive and weak at an early age. Their behavior was unusual—they spent a long time lying on their backs. Approximately fourteen percent of the adult mouse population showed progressive loss of hair, which began at the head and moved down to the middle of the back. Many of the animals died by the sixth month.[9]

If living in Faraday cages, in environments of "reverse pollution" (deprivation of essential electromagnetic waves), has those kinds of adverse effects on animals, what might such conditions do to man? So far, nobody has run laboratory tests, but researchers *have* studied physiological changes in submarine crews— crews surrounded by metal. As A. P. Dubrov reports in *The Geomagnetic Field and Life*:

Despite the life support systems, which eliminate as far as possible any deviations from the norm and allow the crew to stay for a long time under water, considerable disturbances of the functional indices of personnel have been found. For instance, the basal metabolism is lowered, the total leukocyte count in the peripheral blood is reduced and digestive and myogenic leukocytosis is suppressed, the diurnal periodicity of various functions is disturbed, and premorbid states and stomach diseases occur. . . . One can postulate that these disturbances are due to the hypomagnetic environment and the change in the natural background of electromagnetic frequencies.[10]

The fact is, millions of people are now engaged in their own long-term experiments, because many homes in northern climates are, in effect, Faraday cages. A high percentage of the American population is living in homes sheathed in metal siding and insulated with material backed with aluminum foil. The effect is similar to driving under a metal bridge with the car radio on; the sound level drops. Those who choose to live in Faraday cages are perhaps reducing the beneficial effects of the rhythms of the universe, the ancient environment in which man evolved. What the long-term effects will be, if any, is now totally unknown. But that there is at least *some* adverse effect is probable. The conclusion: If householders have a choice, they would be wise to avoid living in houses that act as Faraday cages.

There is another factor, however, that might nullify that advice; under certain conditions a homeowner might do well to isolate himself inside a Faraday cage to *protect* himself. Slowly, man is removing himself from the natural electrical environment, but he is substituting another in its place, this one made by himself—an environment, as the White House council report put it, that is polluted with energy.

Every wire that carries electricity produces electromagnetic waves. And unless you live in a cave, read and cook by flame, and do without radio, TV and telephones, you're surrounded by wires—at home, at work, even in the car. Look at the kinds of equipment found in an average home:

Electric lights
Refrigerator

Radios, TV, and stereo
Clothes washer
Vacuum cleaner
Toaster
Coffeemaker
Mixer
Fry pan
Electric blanket
Air conditioner
Portable heater
Can opener
Clothes dryer
Range
Microwave oven
Water heater
Blender
Hotplate
Dishwasher
Garbage disposal
Infrared lamp
Hair dryer

All of these items produce electromagnetic radiation. Now add to that artificial waves coming in from outside. If high-transmission lines traverse your backyard, or if you're near a radar installation, a microwave relay tower, or an electricity-generating plant, you might be living in electrical soup and not even know it. Every radio station, TV station, and CB unit produces more radiation, and at any given moment most United States citizens are being permeated by many of the country's 1,000 television stations (up from only six in 1945), 8,000 AM and FM radio stations (up from 930 in 1945), and, at last count, 30 million citizen-band radio transmitters (up from nearly zero a decade ago). All told, according to the Environmental Protection Agency, man-made electromagnetic radiation is increasing at the rate of 15 percent a year.[11]

In theory, such radiation has no effect on human beings; the waves pass through or are reflected by living tissue. The theory may or may not be correct. Researchers recently have been questioning the presumption, but as yet no totally conclusive evidence has come to light that such radiation is harmful. (More about this later.) There is, however, a segment of that man-made electrical environment that *is* known to affect human beings, and that is made up of microwaves.

Microwaves lie just below the infrared portion of the electromagnetic spectrum, and they range in wavelength from about 100 centimeters (40 inches) to a millimeter or so (about one twenty-fifth of an inch). The dangers of exposure to high-intensity microwave radiation are not the same as those from exposure to X-rays or nuclear radiation, which can create ionized, internal molecules capable of interfering with or accelerating the division of body cells, and are collectively called "ionizing" radiation. The primary danger from microwaves is thermal— overheating or "cooking" of the cells.

But researchers are becoming increasingly suspicious that there are other, longer-range, insidious effects of microwave radiation that have little to do with heating. If these speculations prove correct, the industrialized world might have a problem of unfathomable complexity on its hands.

Not many years ago, few people had ever heard of microwaves. Today, with the increased use of microwave ovens, and after the famous revelation that the Russians had been focusing microwaves on the American embassy in Moscow, few people haven't. But the radiation involves much more than microwave ovens and bugging. "If you had looked back from space to see the microwave radiation from earth in 1900," says Allan Frey, biophysicist of the Huntington Valley, Pennsylvania, research firm of Randomline, Inc., "the planet would have looked dark. But if you'd look back today, you'd see it glowing like the devil. The stuff is all around us."[12] Dr. John McLaughlin, a radiation specialist in Los Angeles, says that the United States is one "giant microwave oven."[13]

The proliferation of microwaves is enormous, virtually blanketing the nation. Among the many uses of microwaves today that may directly affect the homeowner:

Communications. The first coast-to-coast microwave-relay system for telephones was completed in 1951. Today, more than a quarter million telephone and television relay towers (usually with several generating sources) spiderweb the country.

Radar. Its microwaves blanket areas around all large airports, saturate major harbors and ports (and much of the adjacent shore as well), infuse military installations and the surrounding countryside.

The military. Probably the biggest user of microwave equipment of all is the armed forces. As science writer Paul Brodeur put it in an excellent, two-part 1976 article in *The New Yorker,* "The military has developed an almost insatiable maw for microwave and other electromagnetic devices, employing them in virtually every installation and conveyance it commands."[14]

Satellites. Several communications satellites, which use microwaves to retransmit telephone calls and TV shows, reflect radiation back to earth from hundreds of powerful transmitters (which, even when pointed heavenward, can leak radiation to the sides). Satellites are now being planned that will relay TV shows and messages directly to homeowners' rooftop antennas—and through the houses and their occupants as well.

In the home. Here, microwave devices so far include garage-door openers, burglar-alarm systems, and, of course, the microwave oven.

Sales of microwave ovens in the last few years have skyrocketed, and since 1975 they have exceeded sales of gas ranges. Are they safe? The food they cook is. No harmful substances are known to be produced in food heated by microwaves, and tests show that a larger percentage of germs are destroyed by microwave cooking than by conventional baking.[15] But the question of whether or not the radiation directly harms the chef remains open, mainly because nobody knows for sure the level of microwave exposure that can be considered safe. Yet most experts today agree that unless a quality oven has been damaged (by, for instance, slamming a fork in the door), it likely will leak far below the government-set standard. That may not be low enough. But if the effect of such leakage (and all ovens leak at least a little) is transitory, if the oven is properly maintained so that the door seal doesn't become damaged, and if the chef doesn't habitually watch his dinner being cooked at close range, then the overall health effect is probably less hazardous than that of a conventional, noxious-vapor-producing gas range—at least among chemically sensitive people.

On the other hand, if there are long-range effects of microwave radiation, then we're all in trouble, especially if the use of microwave equipment continues to expand at that 15 percent annual rate. What might be the long-term effects? Again, nobody knows, but a look at the research that *has* been done reveals a series of unnerving facts.

During World War II a Navy-underwritten study of forty-five civilians working with radar revealed that many of the subjects complained of headaches, flushed faces, and eye pain when working near radar equipment. But the report concluded that "no clinical evidence of damage to these personnel" was apparent.[16]

Many of the people who have been exposed disagree. In fact, an organization has been formed, the Radar Victims Network, made up mostly of former radar technicians with ailments they believe were caused by microwaves. Typical is Raymond V. Krabbenhoft, a fifty-four-year-old resident of Sabin, Minnesota, a former Army technician who, during World War II, "was cooked," as he puts it, while repairing radar. His brown hair turned red, he's had three heart attacks and two strokes, he's had several cataracts removed, and he is sterile—all of which he claims resulted from microwave radiation.

The first hard evidence of low-level microwave harm surfaced in the medical press in 1952, after a microwave technician employed by Sandia Corporation in Albuquerque complained to the company's medical director, Frederic G. Hirsh, of "blurred and wavy" vision. Hirsh diagnosed the problem as acute inflammation of the retina, plus seldom-seen bilateral (behind the lens) cataracts. His report of the case ended with the suggestion that it be used "as a means of recalling the attention of ophthalmologists, industrial physicians, and microwave operators to the potentialities of microwave radiation in order that the use of this form of energy will be accompanied by appropriate respect and precautions."[17]

As the years passed, a disproportionate percentage of workers subjected to microwave radiation seemed to be suffering from a whole range of maladies—some minor (irritability, fatigue, "aching eyeballs"), some severe (eye pathology), and some fatal (leukemia, bladder cancer). But because there were no direct tie-ins, and because the observations were not made as part of long-range studies, the reports were described as "inconclusive," or, as in one case, "paradoxical and difficult to interpret."

Meanwhile, the Soviet Union and other Eastern European countries were becoming sufficiently worried about microwave exposures that they were setting safe levels at *one-thousandth* the level deemed acceptable in the United States—an exposure of ten *micro*watts rather then ten *milli*watts per cubic centimeter. They based their concern on a number of long-range, large-scale investigations of human beings and animals. They found, for example, that low-level microwaves affect the central nervous system. They found that long-term, low-level radiation can cause changes in the normal rhythm of brain waves. They found that workers in microwave-rich areas (including radio stations) suffer from a wide variety of neurological problems—overall weakness, vertigo, insomnia, mood changes, and decreased sexual potency.[18] And in Poland, because five cases of birth defects occurred as a result of diathermy treatments, pregnant women today are not allowed to work in occupations where they would be subject to microwaves. In response to the Iron Curtain activities, Professor Charles Susskind, of the University of California's Department of Electrical Engineering, told a Congressional committee:

> We cannot very well dismiss a whole body of scientific literature just because it is Russian. . . . Although ionizing

radiation [such as that produced by radioactive sources] seems to loom larger as a hazard, it would not surprise me in the least if non-ionizing radiation were ultimately to prove a bigger and more vexing problem.[19]

Meanwhile, in this country, other disturbing studies of the effect of low-level microwave radiation on plants and animals have come to light. One, for example, is that they cause chromosome damage, a finding profound in its implications. When New England Institute researchers George Mickey and John H. Heller subjected reproductive cells of fruit flies to pulsed, low-level microwaves, they found that the irradiated flies produced offspring with rough eyes, bristles that appeared singed, strange colors and blistered wings. Why did it happen? Neither Mickey nor Heller can say. The energy levels used were much too low to have caused the mutations by any known means. "The response of the physical scientists . . . was complete bewilderment," says Heller.

> Since my colleagues and I were the ones who initiated this area of scientific activity and since all of our results have since been confirmed elsewhere, I probably have the best overview of anyone in the field. This permits me to state with certainty that I [too] am completely bewildered by the mechanism of action. The phenomena which we have observed seem as impossible (on an energetic basis) as hitting the Empire State Building with a cut-glass fly swatter and having the building crumble. But, it does crumble![20]

The U.S. government has finally become concerned, and today nearly a hundred projects are underway (backed by some $8 million in funding) on the effects of various types of radiation. Meanwhile, the research findings already revealed should be incentive enough to cause anyone who is looking for a new house or a site for a house to avoid microwave-relay towers, ports, airports, and, if possible, even big cities.

Similar to microwaves, but longer in wavelength, is the radiation produced by electrical-power transmission lines. Citizens used to object to the lines simply because the marching towers are eyesores. Today the environmentally sensitive are objecting to them because they could constitute an unfathomable health hazard for those living in homes near them.

Just as in the area of microwaves, few thorough, long-term investigations have been run on physiologically harmful effects of high-voltage transmission lines. However, one series of studies *has* been completed by Andrew Marino of the Syracuse, New York, Veterans Administration Hospital. He reports that (1) directly under the wire, growth is stunted, (2) that from about 30 to 500 feet away, such physiological effects as changes in blood chemistry and electrocardiogram occur, and (3) even as far away as 1,000 feet, "there are behavioral effects, like drops in human reaction time, for instance."[21]

In another study, released in 1969, researchers Nancy Wertheimer and Ed Leeper, of the University of Colorado Medical Center, discovered a possible link between high-current power lines and cancer. They found that children living near large electrical transformers and substations were roughly twice as likely to die from leukemia and nervous-system tumors as those living far from high-power sources.

Robert Becker, the Syracuse V.A. hospital physician, feels that a person living near high-voltage transmission wires is subjected to "chronic stress," and that his body may respond to it in many ways, "from such functional changes as increased irritability and fatigue to such actual pathological states as hypertension and stomach ulcers."[22] Such prolonged stress will enhance the possibility of any weak area of the body developing disease: Heart and kidney stress may lead to hypertension, gastrointestinal stress may bring about ulcers, nervous-system stress may develop into neurosis.

And then there are the common, everyday radio waves. A few years ago scientists believed radio waves had no effect at all on living things. Now they've changed their minds. One experiment that caused the change was conducted by New England Institute's Dr. Heller: He pulsed a shortwave radio signal through a tray containing one-celled paramecia. Ordinarily, the animals swim at random, in all directions. But when Heller beamed the radio waves, the paramecia suddenly began all to move in straight lines, as though in a swimming meet. And when they reached the sides of the container, they flipped over to swim back along the same lines. Why the animals behave in such a strange manner, and what the precise effect of the radio waves on them is, nobody knows. But that there *is* an effect on this one-celled creature is now certain.

What about larger, more complicated animals? Could mammals, for instance, be influenced by such radiation? In order to answer this question, Randomline biophysicist Allan Frey set up an experiment using rats. He placed them in a polystyrene shuttle box divided into two sections, identical except that one lay directly in the beam of a small microwave transmitter. When Frey placed an animal in the box and switched on the transmitter, he discovered that the rat would shuffle off to the nonexposed side and spend about two-thirds of its time there. Frey offers no explanation; the rats should not have known they were being bombarded. But somehow they did. And for some reason they avoided the radiation.[23] Asked one observer: "Do they know something we don't?"

One study conducted by Raytheon's John Osepchuk (mainly to show that microwave ovens aren't so bad after all) concluded that "the television broadcast industry irradiates the country and its population by a factor of more than forty thousand greater than the radiation due to microwave ovens." The Federal Communications Commission has also looked into emissions from TV towers and has come up with figures that show that the radiation level within a one-mile radius of a major TV broadcasting tower can be *ten times* higher than the limit the Soviet Union considers safe for its citizens.

If any doubt lingers that organisms, including human beings, can be influenced by the electrical fields produced by the average home, it should be dispelled by the story of a woman living alone near Santa Barbara, California. She was described as suffering from a number of "nervous" conditions coupled with severe insomnia. She attributed the problem mainly to noises in the house—buzzing, hums, throbs. The electric clock was too loud; the telephone *burred* much of the time; every motor—refrigerator, air conditioner, fan—squealed in its own peculiar voice. The whole house seemed constantly to moan, not loudly, but irritatingly, and it never stopped. Her hearing was ultrasensitive, she concluded, and she decided to do something about the noise. So she called in Clarence Wieska, a member of the Biological Science Department at the University of California at Santa Barbara, a researcher who had done considerable work with electrical noise problems.

Wieska figured that the problem was that some of the house wiring was running across the air-conditioning ducts or some other easily vibrating material, and that the alternating current was causing what is called a 60-Hz sympathetic vibration, a not uncommon problem. So he visited the home with two pieces of equipment: a tape recorder with a pick-up coil in place of the microphone and a sensitive stethoscope.

First he walked from room to room listening, but to him the house seemed to be very quiet. Then he checked all over with his equipment, using the tape recorder to convert the electrical fields so he could hear them through his earphones. "The search coil picked up very strong harmonic frequencies from the 60-cycle electric service, telephone service . . . and metal in the heating system," he wrote later in the journal *Biomedical Sciences Instrumentation*. Then he went back over the stronger electrical-field areas, holding his stethoscope on anything that might be vibrating. He could hear nothing.

But the woman could. "She described the same noise I was hearing on my pickup loop!" he wrote. "The 'impossible deduction' was made that perhaps this woman could hear these alternating current fields without conversion to audible sound waves." To verify the rather strange hypothesis, he conducted a simple test: He unplugged his earphones from the recorder and inserted instead the coil that he had used as a pickup. When he turned the recorder on, he, of course, could hear nothing; no audible sound was coming from the coil. But again, the woman could. "You mean you can't hear that?" she asked, dumbfounded.

While they were discussing the possibilities, the woman suddenly excused herself and answered the telephone. Strange thing, though; it hadn't rung. "For some years the subject at times has been able to answer the phone before it rang," Wieska reported. "The probe was tried during an incoming call and it was found that the phone radiated connection noises just before it rang." Further, the woman told him that she occasionally heard phone conversations when she was near wires, was able to hear recorded music fed into a simple wire loop, and sometimes heard radio stations and high-pitched Morse code in the air.

The woman also said that some homes were much worse than hers, and that she couldn't visit some of her friends because their houses were so noisy (to her) that she could barely hear her friends speak; they were being drowned out by all the background noise. (She had learned over the years to keep such observations to herself.)

After publishing his findings, Wieska received letters from others who were suffering from the same problem. They were all extremely relieved that they finally had been given an explanation—that they actually were *hearing* electromagnetic radiation—and that they were neither alone in their sensitivity nor suffering from some obscure mental problem. One woman told Wieska how happy she was when the electric power went off during storms; it was the only time she found relief from the relentless roar.

"When you consider the electrical makeup of man and the continuously increasing fields we are subjected to," says Wieska, "it seems more reasonable to me that this phenomenon would occur rather than not occur. I believe there could be an increasing incidence rather than an isolated few." And he adds this:

> I recently talked to nurses that had worked in mental institutions. They described patients who were always complaining and trying to get away from the terrible noise. Cotton in their ears did no good, but certain rooms or areas were more quiet for them. I believe that it may be possible that some people may have been driven to these institutions because of the unbearable noise and other effects. . . . Maybe we are putting them in worse field areas. Maybe they could be helped by finding out if they are sensitive, and if they are, placing them in a field-free area may help their condition. I believe this is a vital thing to consider in this age of increasing mental conditions.[24]

The person who can hear electromagnetic radiation is, of course, rare. The point is that if someone can actually *hear* the radiation, the idea of it somehow becomes more real—not theory, not simply curving lines on graphs. The waves are real and so are their influences, even though nobody knows for certain just what those influences are. But as that White House council stated in its final report, "The consequences of undervaluing or misjudging the biological effects of long-term, low-level exposure could become a critical problem for the public health, especially if genetic effects are involved."

Which, to the homeowner, all boils down to the prudence of selecting a home as far from strong radiation sources as possible—with some specific suggestions presented in Chapter 8.

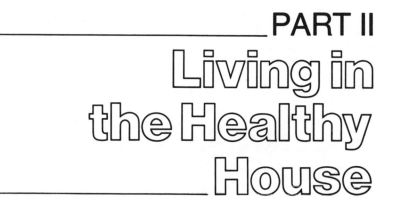

PART II

Living in the Healthy House

6

Clothing and Furnishings

A house should be a sanctuary, a refuge, a place for relaxation, for rest. It should be a place of safety, sheltering the inhabitants from the forces of nature, shielding them from the antagonistic world outside. It should be what it was to our ancestors: a cocoon of protection; there are no thorns in a house, no storms, no stinging insects, no preying animals.

In modern, industrialized, "civilized" societies, few houses are like that. They do keep out the rain and insects, do provide comfortable temperatures, do provide a place to hide from the world. But in matters of health, the average house is the enemy, filled with noxious particles, virulent chemicals, alien radiation.

Part I of this book dealt with principles and identified environmental hazards. In the following chapters, we will apply those principles to the components of the home to show specifically how the house can be used as a tool for maintaining health, rather than remaining, as it does throughout Western society, a major cause of illness.

Many people still think of the field of medicine as being centered around *curing,* with relatively little thought given to *prevention.* Yet finding and avoiding causes of illness is obviously more intelligent than treating the effects. And the fact is, prevention of illness is not all that difficult. When one considers the range of potential problems described in the preceding chapters, he might feel like one of my recent patients, who said, "You've taken away my favorite foods, thrown out my furniture, stripped me of makeup, and sealed me away from the world. I might as well slit my throat and get it over with." Actually, a *radical* change of life-style is rarely necessary. A situation that may catastrophically affect one person may not bother another environmentally sensitive person at all. And nobody is susceptible to *all* facets of his environment. Often even the extremely sensitive person can avoid the source of his problem without too much trouble, and if he does so successfully, an accidental exposure might produce a severe reaction, but one that's *temporary*. Further, if a reaction to a particular chemical effector is not overwhelming, simple avoidance of massive doses might be enough. And because many substances act only in concert with others (mold, for example, may not be a problem with a specific person except when coupled with ragweed pollen), the elimination of one may make the avoidance of another unnecessary.

A logical place to begin is with the immediate surroundings: clothing and furnishings.

Clothing

Apparently, nearly everything that human beings place next to their skin, from shoes to jewelry, makes some people suffer in one way or another. Usually the problem is an allergic reaction, but with the exception of wool (which often causes dermatitis, acting as a combination allergen and a simple physical irritant), most clothing problems are caused not by the materials themselves, but by what is in them. And although many people believe that the biggest troublemaker is the dye, that rarely is the case. Today's dyes are chemically linked so tightly to material that even highly sensitive individuals can tolerate them.

The biggest problem with clothing, I've found, comes not from the manufacturing processes, but from the home laundry room. Bleaches, detergents, anti-hard-water agents, presoaks, fabric softeners, antistatic agents—all can lead to skin problems of various kinds because of the small quantities of these chemicals usually remaining in the garment. (See Chapter 7 for relatively harmless laundry products.)

Problems with clothing chemicals don't always begin in the laundry, however. Not long ago a man came in with sore and itching feet the color of cherries. We traced the cause to his shoes. He was sensitive to the adhesive that bound the canvas lining to the leather. Such adhesive contains two substances that can lead to reactions: antioxidants and accelerators.

On another occasion, a woman brought in her seven-year-old twins, both of whom were suffering from general itching around their necks and over most of their legs and arms. Because it was November, the cause here was easy to identify. Early the previous spring, when the mother had packed the woolen snowsuits away, she had sprinkled them with a good helping of mothballs. When the children put the winter clothing on again, both developed dermatitis where the snowsuits came in contact with their skin. Removal of such mothproofing contamination is not easy; it may take a year or two to air out, although cleaning can speed the process.

Some answers are considerably more elusive. One patient with a severe rash across his forehead puzzled me until I happened to notice that he was carrying a cap. The problem apparently was the interior leather band. Chromium (commonly used in the rapid-tanning process) in leather in hats and caps often causes reactions, and in this case, when the patient stopped wearing his hat, his symptoms disappeared.

Two other unsuspected clothing irritants: the rubber in bras and elastic-topped underwear, and the nickel or other metal in foundation garments.

I'm often asked about the difference between synthetic and natural fibers for sensitive persons. I tend to prefer natural products, even though many people react adversely to some of them, particularly to wool. The reason, I've found, is that patients react to natural products either significantly or not at all, whereas with synthetics, a reaction might be so low-level it isn't noticed, and yet it may, year after year, contribute to an overall lowered efficiency. (Generally, the less odor a synthetic fabric has, the less likely it is to cause reactions. Nylon and rayon have been reported to be superior to most other woven synthetic materials, including Orlon and Dacron.)

In addition, synthetics tend to hold electrical charges when worn. Pull a dress of synthetic fabric over your head on a cold, dry day, and the charge generated by the friction causes it to stick to your body. (On a humid day, the moisture in the air helps conduct the charge to earth.) The presence of a charge is thought to be physiologically burdensome to the wearer. In *The Ion Effect*, Fred Soyka tells of a girl in London who at the age of fourteen began "to suffer from severe migraine because of clothing— then cured it herself." As she entered adolescence, she began to wear nylon bras and panties, and she also started to suffer severe headaches for the first time in her life.

> When she graduated to slips and nightdresses and pretty nylon blouses, she became a full-fledged migraine sufferer. Her local general practitioner could offer neither explanation nor help beyond suggesting the onset of menstruation as a cause. But the girl was bright enough to associate the clothes of blooming womanhood with her problem and abandoned the feminine underwear and nightdresses. Now her clothes are of cotton, which is the only fiber that creates no charge at all, and of natural fibers like wool, which carry little charge of either kind.[1]

Furnishings

Before his life has run its course, the average man will spend nearly a quarter of a century in bed. As a physician, if I knew I was going to be anywhere for that length of time, I'd ask myself, How will this place affect me? Is it a healthy environment in which to spend that much time? Obvious questions. And yet almost nobody considers the health aspects of the bedroom.

Strictly from a health viewpoint, the ideal sleeping quarters would contain nothing but the bed—no upholstered furniture, no rugs, no stuffed toys, no drapes, because all of these generate housedust of various sorts. That large, relaxing chair, that comfortable sofa, *any* overstuffed furniture should be replaced, if need be, with furniture of modern Danish or similar design. The new items should be of simple lines, using stuffings of synthetic fibers instead of cotton, kapok, or animal hair. Cellulose padding should be especially avoided; the breakdown products are cellulose particles and dust mites—both major problem sources.

No furniture polish or wax should ever be used on either the furniture or the floor. Finishes should be hard, and they should require no maintenance except washing. In fact, before you place a new (or newly refinished) piece of furniture in the bedroom, it's a good idea to "season" it somewhere else in the house to make sure that the finish has thoroughly dried, that all noxious elements have evaporated. Hard plastic finishes on furniture and floors are especially good, except when sunlight falls directly on them for prolonged periods. Strong sunlight may enhance depolymerization, the gradual breakdown of the plastic surface, a process that produces *monomers,* or molecules of less complicated chemical makeups. They become airborne, and although the quantity is small enough that they rarely become a problem, monomers do add to the total petrochemical pollution in a home's atmosphere.

If possible, clothing should be kept in dressers and closets in adjacent rooms, not where you sleep. If you don't, even if you keep drawers and closet doors tightly shut, when you open them the room becomes bathed in a snowstorm of invisible dust and vapors.

Mattresses, box springs, and pillows should be encased in special dustproof covers, products designed specifically to be inert; ordinary plastic casings—the kind most department stores carry—probably *aren't* inert, and they well could produce tiny amounts of noxious vapors for months, even for years, which could lead to acute sensitivity. (See Appendix C for suppliers of acceptable products.) Before use, any casing should be aired for a few days—in the sun, if possible. If you select a polyurethane or foam-rubber mattress, or pillows stuffed with Dacron or Acrilan, no casings are needed. Many people, however, are sensitive to polyurethane or sponge rubber and do better with a Dacron-filled spring mattress. Unfortunately, there's no way to predict, and trial and error can be expensive. But if you can get a sample of the material and sleep with it under or near you, you may be able to see whether or not you're sensitive.

A person highly sensitive to housedust should also remove pennants and pictures from the bedroom walls, along with mirrors (unless flush-mounted), magazines, books, and bookshelves. All are dust catchers, and all can hinder cleaning. All storage—on shelves or under the bed —should be removed too.

Window shades should also be eliminated; they are excellent dust catchers. Even the flexible-plastic, washable type are poor—particularly those exposed to direct sunlight—because of the vapors. (And they usually smell for months.) Drapes, of course, are out. Venetian blinds, because they too are dust catchers, should be cleaned often; otherwise, when you open the window the breeze will envelop you in a housedust fog.

Bedspreads, blankets, sheets, and pillowcases should be of well-washed (and well-rinsed) cotton. Some sheets, particularly the drip-dry, no-iron variety, have been subjected to a plasticized starch treatment that is not removable by laundering. If you are troubled by reactions from some sheets and not others, this might be the reason. Give the treated sheet to some less sensitive person. In any case, all bedclothes should be washable. Dry-cleaning establishments do some strange things with blankets (such as treating them with chlorinated hydrocarbons or failing to thoroughly remove cleaning compounds), and you'll be safer cleaning blankets yourself.

Electric blankets should be avoided by the chemically susceptible because the heat tends to drive off plastic monomers from the material and vapors from internal rubber cases. In addition, even though the effect of sleeping night after night in an alternating electromagnetic field is unknown, it seems to me too much of a gamble. I prefer an extra blanket.

I suspect that highly sensitive patients may benefit from a *nonmetallic* bed. I know of no evidence that sleeping in the proximity of metal is detrimental, but it is possible that an iron bed could influence whatever electromagnetic waves are present—either blocking natural radiation or concentrating man-made waves. Only recently has metal been cheap enough to be employed in beds; our immediate ancestors slept on wood, and ancient man used the ground. On the remote chance that a metal bed might have some influence, I have installed beds in my home with flexible wooden slats instead of metal springs. (Such beds are commercially available.)

The rules for bedrooms apply to the rest of the house as well, even though the importance isn't so great. Carried to a logical extreme, the ideal healthy house would be devoid of everything—furniture, carpets, bric-a-brac, books, magazines, pictures. Not only would such a house be healthy, but it would be easy to clean. Obviously, nobody—even the most sensitive person—is going to live in an empty house, but a good approach is to think of ways to furnish one's house more simply, then compromise as desirable for convenience and aesthetic reasons.

One area in which there should be little compromise for the highly sensitive person, however, is floors. And in particular, carpets and their padding. Carpets have a multitude of disadvantages. Among them:

• They entrap housedust, and when you walk across them you're followed by a housedust smog. Even a freshly vacuumed carpet remains a repository of an amazing quantity of housedust. You can prove this to yourself by thoroughly vacuuming a corner of a carpet, then folding the corner over a piece of white paper and tapping the backing. Your paper will no longer be white.

• Carpets *generate* housedust and often noxious vapors as well. Whether they are made of vegetable fiber (cotton, jute, coconut, linen, silk) or synthetics (acrylic, nylon, rayon, polyester, polypropylene) or animal hair (wool, blends of goat, cow, horse, pig), normal wear will cause microscopic bits of the material to break off and become airborne, adding a huge volume of particles to the home air pollution. And in winter, as the microscopic bits of synthetic carpet circulate through the heating system, they burn, change their chemistry, and add an unbelievable variety of strange and alien vapors to the air. A burning synthetic may produce a hundred or more compounds, from sulfuric acid to hydrogen cyanide.[2] Trapped in the closed environment of a winter home, such compounds may be breathed and rebreathed by the occupants for months.

• New carpets often arrive permeated with insecticides, and they waft their poisons through the house indefinitely. Just when the vapors begin to decrease somewhat, the rug is ready for professional cleaning— and it often returns soaked with insecticide again. Rugs sent out for cleaning should be accompanied by a note demanding that no mold inhibitors, mothproofing materials, or dirt-repellent coatings be used.

• In wintertime, a person walking across a rug generates charges that disrupt the electrostatic environment.

So, if possible, eliminate floor coverings entirely, particularly wall-to-wall carpets, which are virtually impossible to clean. Throw rugs, however, are not so bad, if they are small enough to fit into the washing machine. Braided rugs are preferable. Pile rugs are all right only if the pile is short: High-pile rugs collect more dust and may be a repository for mold as well.

Furniture coverings also require some thought. The best material is natural fibers, such as cotton and wool (unless a sensitivity to wool has been established). Soft sheet-plastic covers are to be avoided because of the vapors given off, although Naugahyde seems to be tolerable even to some sensitive individuals. Stuffed furniture is to be avoided; however, if you do want it, avoid kapok and cotton batting, because such materials generate house-dust. Consider instead furniture stuffed with high-quality polyester, such as Dacron (Dupont) or Kodel (Eastman Kodak). Some lesser-quality polyesters have been reported to be irritating to sensitive patients. Foam rubber and polyurethane stuffing are less desirable choices; of the two, polyurethane is probably the lesser of the two evils, but both should be avoided if possible.

To recapitulate, the accompanying table lists textiles used for floor covering, clothing, and furniture, along with their appropriateness for a healthy house.

The floors themselves, throughout the house, should be of some chemically inert material. In addition to hard-wood surfaced with polyurethane (applied during the summer months when the windows can be opened, and preferably just before a vacation), nonporous ceramic tile is an excellent choice. Glazed ceramic and surfaced hardwood offer four main advantages over other floor coverings:

1. They hold virtually no electric charges, in contrast with carpets and plastic surfaces.
2. They are inert; they generate neither airborne particles nor gases.
3. They require no waxing.
4. They are easily cleaned of dust.

Also shown is a tabular summary of various floor coverings used in homes.

The interior walls of a healthy house can be of natural wood or they can be painted (see Chapters 7 and 9 for specific suggestions), but they shouldn't be wallpapered. For one thing, wallpaper paste frequently contains anti-insect and antimold chemicals that can contaminate the environment. The same chemicals are often impregnated in the wallpaper itself, and even though the long-term effects of breathing such vapors has not been established, the practice raises such obvious questions that the sensitive individual (and probably everyone else as

TEXTILES USED IN THE HOME

BASIC SUBSTANCE	TRADE NAMES	USES	COMMENTS
NATURAL SUBSTANCES			
Animal products			
Wools/Silk		Blankets, draperies, rugs, upholstery	Hair from sheep, goat, camel, etc., and silk from silkworm cocoons. Good choice, unless allergy has been established.
Vegetable products			
Cotton		Same as above	Cellulose from cotton plant. Good choice.
Linen			Cellulose from flax plant. Good choice.
Mineral			
Glass (fiberglass)	Fiberglas Beta PPG Uniglas	Wallpaper, draperies	Silica sand, limestone, aluminum, borax. There is a danger in washing fiberglass curtains with clothes; tiny spicules of glass break off and embed themselves in the clothing; when the clothing is worn, an extremely irritating dermatitis can develop. Run machine through complete cycle after washing fiberglass. There is also a possibility that glass may break off from fiberglass draperies and, aerosolized, be breathed by the occupants of the room. Therefore, fiberglass is low on the list of choices for drapes.
SYNTHETIC SUBSTANCES			
Cellulose			
Acetate	Acele Celanese Avisco	Bedspreads, drapes, rugs, upholstery, curtains	Sensitive people usually prefer natural fibers to synthetic. If you can verify that you don't react, then these choices might be accept-

Regener- ated cellulose	Rayon Cupion Enka Fortisan	Blankets, draperies, rugs, tablecloths, curtains	able in limited quantity. Remember that synthetics hold a charge and contribute to electrostatic pollution.
Polyamide	Nylon Nylon 501 Caprolan Cumuloft Nylon 6 Antron	Bedspreads, rugs, upholstery	
Olefins	Herculon Ethylene Vectra	Blankets, rugs Upholstery, webbing	
Polyesters Dihydric alcohol and terepha- thalic	Dacron Kodel Fortrel	Bedding, curtains, draperies, upholstery	

FLOOR AND SURFACE COVERINGS

MATERIAL	CONTENT	COMMENTS
Ceramic	Concrete, stone, brick, tile	Best choice, especially for sleeping quarters: no electric charge problem, easy to clean (no wax necessary) if sufficiently hard, nonporous tile is selected—dense quarry or glazed. Some porous tiles require waxing; avoid them.
Cellulose Wood	Hardwoods: oak, birch, beach, maple, pecan, teak, walnut	Good choice if covered with polyurethane. (Finish in summer months only.) Polyurethane wears well and resists water.

FLOOR AND SURFACE COVERINGS *(cont.)*

	Softwoods: pine, spruce, cedar.	Not a suitable choice for a floor because they're resinous and produce petrochemical problems. (They also wear poorly.)
Cork tile	Cork particles compressed and heated with petrochemical binders	Attractive, but is a petrochemical polluter. Avoid.
Linoleum	Wood dust, cork particles, pigments, gums, and linseed oil compressed into burlap or felt	High potential for pollution because of composition and because such floors are commonly waxed to retain sheen. Avoid. Choose a more durable, less potentially troublesome product.
Plastic Vinyl tiles and sheets	Pigments, plasticizers, vinyl plus fillers molded with heat and pressure	The petrochemical problem has been obviated by the coating of vinyl, but plastic holds an electrical charge, producing electrostatic pollution. In addition, sunlight falling on surface may cause monomer-vapor pollution.
Vinyl-asbestos tile.	Fibers (asbestos, cotton, others), vinyl-plastic resins	
Asphalt tile	Fibers (asbestos, cotton, others), pigments, plasticizers, resins	Easy to clean, but holds electric charge. Most products need waxing; some don't. If this floor is selected, a nonwaxing type is mandatory.
Rubber	Rubber (natural or synthetic)	Rubber is not tolerable by petrochemically sensitive people.

---

well) should shun them. On the other hand, wallpapers applied with paste that *doesn't* contain antimold chemicals could be a good source of mold spores, and if one consistently breathes mold spores, he can easily develop a sensitivity. Fabric "wallpapers" add another worry:

The surface can break down and produce a cellulose-dust problem. And wallpapers coated with plastic film for easy washing hold electric charges, which intensify electrostatic pollution.

Furnishing the house with items that promote health rather than illness presents fewer problems than one might expect. The key word for this chapter is *clean*, applied with both meanings: clean, as in the elimination of dust and odors; clean, as in simple lines.

Maintaining the Healthy House

You can do little about certain of the things that may be making your house unhealthy. If you live in the path of microwave-relay towers, if thermal inversions over your city turn the air into an atmospheric sewer, if your valley suffers from the local equivalent of the foehn winds, then your best move is to do just that. And confronted by the ever-expanding list of man-made chemicals—one new substance synthesized by the American industry every *minute* [1]—the odds against living a healthy life seem overwhelming. But the situation isn't actually that bad. If you eat well, avoid worthless or excessive medication, choose the chemicals that you bring into the home carefully, and maintain the house sensibly, your body will probably have enough cellular energy in reserve to fight the alien chemicals and radiation you can't avoid.

Once you have eliminated the worst of the household polluters, maintaining a relatively healthy environment is mostly a matter of *awareness*, of keeping in mind the environmental villains over which you have the most control.

Particles

The main way to maintain a low-housedust condition is, of course, by frequent cleaning. A few suggestions:

Don't use dusters, mops, or brooms (they scatter dust), and certainly no commercial dusting oils or other fume-producing preparations. Move all furniture to the center of the room when you clean, so you can reach the corners, and with a damp rag wipe moldings, light fixtures, shelves, and door and window tops. The bedroom of an allergen-sensitive person, in particular, should be kept scrupulously clean, with frequent washings of floors, walls, ceilings, and bedsprings. If the sufferer is a child, he should, of course, be sent out to play. And throw open the windows to breeze away the dust you raise, particularly when vacuuming. (In winter, wear a coat if you have to.)

Vacuum cleaners present a peculiar problem. They're by far the most effective device for removing dust, and yet most of them pollute more than they clean; they suck in dust from surfaces, then blow the smaller particles through the filter or bag into the air, particles that, because of their very small size, may slide through the body's filtering mechanisms to lodge deep in the lungs. The best vacuum system is one built into the house, a system that pulls dust into a central unit, then blows it *outside*. (Specialized equipment, if prescribed by your allergist, may be used as a medical tax deduction.) Short of this ideal, a second choice is the Rainbow vacuum cleaner (see Appendix C-Manufacturers' List). It uses water as a filter and is better than most vacuum cleaners in not polluting the air with dust particles.

The question of whether windows should be open or closed during the summer depends on the inhabitants of the house. Unless your home nestles in an industrial smog or lies next to a truck route, chances are that the air inside the house is much more polluted than that outside. So throw wide the windows to flush out your house, and keep them open in comfortable weather—unless a family member has a pollen allergy that is in season. Then you'll have to experiment. Perhaps it would be acceptable to open windows only on the downwind side of the house. Or perhaps windows could be opened in the very early morning or at night, when pollen production is usually lowest.

Or provide a room air conditioner—creating an island of escape—and keep the windows open throughout the rest of the house. Most air conditioners have built-in filters, and because no outside air is brought inside (unless the unit is specially adjusted to do so), the pollen stays out and the housedust gradually diminishes. An air conditioner does tend to remove negative ions from the room, however. And many people are adversely affected by the sudden temperature changes encountered when entering or leaving an air-conditioned area.

A simpler device for removing airborne particles is a forced-air filtering unit, essentially a fan that blows the air through a filter. Paper filters are especially efficient because their effectiveness actually increases as they are used; as the layers of dust are laid down on the inexpensive paper medium, the dust itself acts as a screening mechanism, filtering out smaller and smaller particles until completely clogged. Maintenance is easy; the paper is discarded. Avoid filters sprayed with a sticky substance supposedly designed to trap particles. The efficiency is low, and the sticky material will volatilize.

Although forced-air heating systems with built-in filters are excellent removers of airborne housedust, most people find that running an air-circulation system through the summer is counterproductive. The units do remove dust, but because the ductwork is made of metal, they also eliminate negatively charged ions, resulting in an electrically unhealthful atmosphere. And at present, there is no satisfactory mechanical method of replacing those lost ions. I do *not* recommend ion generators. All, to my knowledge, give off ozone (although some companies dispute this), and ozone is toxic. The small benefit that would result from the additional air ions produced would probably be more than offset by adverse effects of the ozone, even though the quantity is small.

Running a heating or air-conditioning system without the proper filter, of course, is most detrimental; it keeps the housedust in constant motion, and airborne.

One filtration system that should be avoided entirely is the electrostatic kind. These devices pull the air through two electrically charged grids, one positive, one negative. As dust particles pass, they stick to one or the other, depending on their charge. Such systems are effective—they remove some ninety percent of the airborne particles—but they have four disadvantages: (1) They're relatively expensive. (2) They require frequent cleaning; unlike passive filters, they become increasingly inefficient between cleanings because as the grids become coated with dust, their ability to attract additional dust decreases. (3) They discharge ozone. True, the amount produced is very small, but *none* is better than some. (4) They neutralize ions, reducing the ionic level of the environment, the opposite of what is desirable. (If you already use an electrostatic filter in your heating system, perhaps your unit has space to add a second collecting cell. A filter of activated charcoal added downstream from the electrostatic filter will eliminate part of the trouble; at least it will collect the ozone before it is blown into your living area.)

Mold

Mold forms where it's damp, and there are more damp places in your home than you probably realize. The obvious place to start a mold-eradication program is in the basement. Most basements are at least a little damp, and most produce spores by the millions that gradually float upstairs to waft throughout the house.

The first thing to do, of course, is to throw out all those old, damp piles of material you've been storing in the basement and elsewhere—newspapers, books, magazines, carpets, overstuffed furniture, pillows. Clothes waiting to be laundered sometimes produce mold, as do clothes washed but not yet dried. And sleeping bags should always be aired out thoroughly after use.

An additional source of mold is a humidifier, built-in or standing. The solution here is to clean it frequently, perhaps once a week, with a stiff vegetable scrub brush. Some manufacturers recommend that detergent be used, or a bacterial deterrent, or even household bleach—all extremely poor ideas because the chemicals will be aerosolized and breathed by the inhabitants of the home throughout the six-month heating season. Use only water.

Basements that are only occasionally damp often can be controlled by dehumidifiers. I recommend buying the largest-capacity model available, one equipped with a control that automatically turns it off when the humidity drops to an acceptable level. Because most people spend little time in the basement, the level can be considerably lower than would be comfortable in the rest of the house.

If the basement seems to become more damp after a rain, the most frequent cause is simply that the roof downspout is depositing water too near the foundation. The quick solution, of course, is to extend the leader to carry the water away and downhill. Sometimes, however, a more complex solution is necessary: Foundation drains must be installed. (See Chapter 9 for design suggestions.)

The two other mold-producing areas of the house are, not surprisingly, the bathroom and the kitchen. In the bath, a favorite place for mold to grow is in the grouting between tiles and caulking between the tub and the wall. Check to see that the caulking or grouting is still intact; if not, repair. Shower curtains are another common bathroom mold producer (especially if they are of the lined type), as is the floor at the rear base of the toilet. The solution to an overall bathroom mold problem is air circulation, and almost all bathroom troubles can be solved with a built-in shower exhaust.

In the kitchen, mold frequently develops at the sink-wall junction and around the bottom of the cold-water pipe. A small amount of borax—a natural antimold agent —sprinkled over the area will usually solve the problem. A particularly bad mold source is the surplus-water tray on self-defrosting refrigerators. You may not even know you have one. Reach under the bottom and see. Use borax here too. A kitchen wall vent will blow away mold spores, and odors and vapors as well.

I'm often asked if houseplants are a cause of allergic reactions. The answer is yes, but not because of the pollen; houseplants rarely produce any. It's the mold growing on the soil surfaces. A layer of crushed stone on the surface will, to some extent, inhibit mold dispersal.

Vapors

The two prime sources of noxious vapors in the home are evaporating chemicals and heating and cooking equipment. The worst fuel is gas; a healthy house should not even be connected to a gas line. If you are cooking with gas now, I urge you in the strongest terms possible to switch over as quickly as practical to electricity.

If you are *heating* with gas or oil and suspect that you might be sensitive, I suggest that if your system is of the forced-hot-air type, you have someone from the gas company or from your oil-burner service agency perform tests to see if the firebox is leaking. (The firebox is the combustion chamber of the furnace. The air flows around but not into it, to be warmed before passing into the living area.) The tests must be performed using instrumentation (Bacharach or equal test equipment); tests performed by using the sense of smell—by placing an odoriferous substance into the firebox—are inadequate. If you are heating with oil, check every so often to see that no oil is leaking from line junctions, and be sure the furnace is adjusted by a professional at least once a year.

In addition, I suggest that you may want to close your furnace off from the rest of the house if possible, and plan eventually to change over to heating equipment of a more environmentally compatible nature. (For a fuller discussion, see Chapter 9.)

One other thing you might consider is *outside venting* for your furnace—the use of an outside source of air, instead of air from the furnace room, for combustion. The reason is that air *directly* heated by the flame is not circulated, but in turn heats water pipes or a reservoir (in hot-water systems), or an air chamber (in hot-air systems), then goes up the chimney. A typical burner may require 2,000 or 3,000 cubic feet of air an hour, and that air must come from somewhere; without an outside vent, it comes in mainly through cracks around doors and windows. (If the basement or furnace room is well caulked, insulated, and sealed, burner efficiency suffers.)

An outside source of furnace air, experts say, not only saves an average of about 15 percent on fuel bills, but results in a more healthful humidity level in the house.*

One particularly vexing vapor question is that involving wall paints. The only really safe thing to say is that with any finish, apply it only in the spring or early summer, and with the windows wide open. Let the house air as long as possible before being closed in for the winter. Beyond that, guidelines for finishes are hard to draw; the paint industry uses more than 600 ingredients, and the difficulty of predicting the health effects on the consumer is overwhelming. And the fact is, no clear-cut evidence exists that any type is better physiologically than any other—although there have been a few clinical observations:

Casein paints rarely cause adverse reactions, even among the chemically sensitive. However, because casein is a milk derivative, it will support mold growth in moist areas, such as the bathroom and kitchen.

Latex paints are not recommended, mainly because the odor has been reported to persist for many months, and the fumes have been held responsible for perpetuating chronic illnesses.[2]

Alkyd-base paints seem to be the best tolerated. (Alkyd is a contraction for alkyl and acid, two ingredients.) Besides the usual household variety, it also comes in a special "odorless" type.

Epoxy paints are excellent regarding durability. But they take an exceptionally long time to dry and should be avoided unless the painted surface can be aged for three to six months before bringing it into the home. This virtually eliminates these paints for use on walls.

---

* For a discussion of do-it-yourself installation, see Evan Powell, "Outside Venting Can Trim Your Fuel Bills," *Popular Science*, December 1978, p. 116.

The problem of toxic vapors from evaporating chemicals is a never-ending one for the conscientious householder. Most of the other common agents that give trouble are covered in the accompanying maintenance guide.

HOUSEHOLD MAINTENANCE GUIDE

PURPOSE	AVOID	SUBSTITUTE
I. CLEANING AGENTS		
Laundry bleach	Chlorine-containing	Oxygen (nonchlorine) bleaches. Example: Polytex liquid & Clorox II, which contains hydrogen peroxide; others contain perborate.
Laundry whitener		*Miracle White (Beatrice Food Co., Chicago 60632)
Laundry detergent	Complex chemicals	Basic L (Shaklee Co.), SA8 (Amway Co.)
Antihardwater agents		Calgon (use only if your water is hard).
Presoaks		Omit these products temporarily and try them later, if you need them, to see if they cause a problem.
Fabric softeners and anti-static agents		As above
Scouring powder	Chlorinated products	Bon Ami
Dishwasher compound	Complex chemicals	Basic D (Shaklee Co.) Automatic Dishwasher Detergent, Dishdrops (Amway Co.)

*Contains chemicals that may not be tolerated by some individuals.
**Poisonous.

HOUSEHOLD MAINTENANCE GUIDE (cont.)

PURPOSE	AVOID	SUBSTITUTE
General household	Complex chemicals	LOC, regular or high suds (Amway), Basic H (Shaklee), Basic I (Shaklee). For heavy-duty cleaning, sodium bicarbonate (Arm & Hammer *Baking* Soda), sodium *carbonate*** (Arm & Hammer *Washing* Soda-Sal Soda), trisodium phosphate.** (Wear rubber gloves.)
Window cleaner	Ammonia-containing window sprays	Vinegar (one tablespoon to a quart of water), Bon Ami Cake Soap, borax
Disinfectant	Those containing phenol, creosol (read label)	Borax, sodium carbonate (Arm & Hammer Washing Soda-Sal Soda)
Mold inhibitor		*Zephiran concentrate: one oz./gallon of distilled water. Acts as a fungicide and general germicide. Available in drugstores. Preferred: borax, a natural bleach, useful in washing clothes; it is a natural antimold agent as well. Sprinkle in moldy places to retard growth.
Bar soap		Bon Ami Cake, Ivory, Lowilla
Grease-spot remover	Organic solvents	Sprinkle fuller's earth on the spot; it absorbs the grease like a sponge in fifteen minutes to two hours. (Careful with colored fabrics; they may lighten if left too long.)

*Contains chemicals that may not be tolerated by some individuals.
**Poisonous.

Rug cleaner		Procter and Gamble's Orvus Extra Granules or Orvus NWA Paste
Chromium cleaner	Complex chemicals	(1) Pure cider vinegar and a soft cloth; polish with a paper towel. (2) Whiting (calcium carbonate), available at paint stores. Use on a damp cloth; dry with a soft cloth.
Sterling-silver cleaner	Complex chemicals	(1) Whiting on a damp cloth. (2) Soapy solution of baking soda and water. (3) "Electrolyte method": cream of tartar (from drugstore or supermarket) or sodium bicarbonate, one teaspoon in a quart of warm water. Use an aluminum pan or put aluminum foil into the solution. Let the silver soak in the solution until shiny.
Brass, bronze, copper, and steel cleaner	Complex chemicals	Dampen fine table salt with vinegar or lemon juice; rub.
Room deodorants	Avoid all commercial products.	An electric fan to blow air out of a musty room or closet. Borax, as a natural deodorant and antimold agent. Sprinkle it in the corners.
Heavy scouring	Steel-wool pads impregnated with soap	Plain steel wool and separate soap cake (use a tolerated soap).

*Contains chemicals that may not be tolerated by some individuals.
**Poisonous.

HOUSEHOLD MAINTENANCE GUIDE (*cont.*)

PURPOSE	AVOID	SUBSTITUTE
Furniture polish	Commercial furniture polish	Olive oil, pure (100%), lemon oil, beeswax, beeswax and olive oil, raw (*not* boiled) linseed oil (may be allergenic). The tackiness of vegetable and animal oils will disappear with much rubbing.
Crayon-mark remover	Commercial solvents	Plain vinegar. Apply sparingly and rub. Let dry. Follow with fuller's earth.
Gum, tar remover	Commercial solvents	To remove from skin, hair: Use smooth peanut butter, vegetable oil, or Crisco, followed by soap and water.

II. ANTI-INSECT PROGRAM

Roaches	Petro-chemical insecticides	Powdered boric acid.** Slow-acting but sure.
		Roach Prufe (Copper Brite, Inc., 5147 W. Jefferson Blvd., Los Angeles, CA 90016)
		TAT roach trap** for German roaches, Harris roach tablet** for oriental and large American roaches and silverfish. A powder made of 70% flour, 10% sugar (confectioner's 10X), 10% cocoa powder, and 10% boric acid or borax.** (Don't use if you have small children or animals.) Gator Roach Traps contain arsenic (DeSoto Chemical Co., Inc., Arcadia, FL).**

*Contains chemicals that may not be tolerated by some individuals.
**Poisonous.

Ants	Petro-chemical insecticides	TAT ant trap.** Honey/boric acid mixture.**
Fleas	Petro-chemical insecticides	Diatomaceous earth (obstructs insects' breathing apparatus). Pyrethrum. Rotenone.
Ticks	Petro-chemical insecticides	Silica gel (careful not to inhale). Ticks will loosen hold if touched by a drop of tincture of merthiolate.[3]
Moths	Moth flakes, mothballs, moth spray, mothproof shelf paper	Brush clothes (eggs are fragile and are destroyed). Hang out on line for air and sunlight every two weeks to a month. Avoid grease spots; have clothes dry-cleaned. Seal in airtight containers. Freeze in deep freeze to kill larvae.

A natural recipe used by Chicago-area weavers and spinners:

Rosemary	½ lb.
Mint	½ lb.
Thyme	¼ lb.
Ginseng (optional)	¼ lb.
Cloves	2 tbs.

Mix and put in cheesecloth bags for use similar to a sachet.

Termites	Chlordane and other "soil-poisoning" methods	Mineral insecticides: copper chromate, cryolite.** Discuss old methods of using these materials with county extension agent or exterminator. For prevention, Wolmanized pressure-treated wood (see Chapter 9); build correctly in the first place.

*Contains chemicals that may not be tolerated by some individuals.
**Poisonous.

HOUSEHOLD MAINTENANCE GUIDE (*cont.*)

PURPOSE	AVOID	SUBSTITUTE
Wallpaper	Mold and insect inhibitor	Borax or boric acid, one tablespoon to quart of starch paste to make antimold and anti-insect paste.** Nothing is both safe and mold- or insectproof. Best to avoid wallpaper entirely.
Fly control	Insecticide strips	Flypaper.

III. MISCELLANEOUS

PURPOSE	AVOID	SUBSTITUTE
Glue		Glue Bird or Elmer's brands
Lubrication	Machine oils	Graphite (check with manufacturer before using). Light mineral oil (medicinal grade, from pharmacies) may be tolerable. Motors requiring no lubrication at all are preferred.
Shoe and boot waterproofing	Synthetic, odoriferous preparations	Peccard leather waterproofing products (Peccard Chemical Co., Inc., 1836 Industrial Drive, Green Bay, WI 54302)
Heat/air-conditioning system filters	Oil- or hexachlorophene-impregnated	Untreated filters, preferably paper
Fireplace chimneys		Keep damper closed when not in use and have cleaned at end of season to stop soot from filtering into home.
Volatile solvents and terpenes	Avoid in all forms	

*Contains chemicals that may not be tolerated by some individuals.
**Poisonous.

Notes on Household Maintenance Guide

1. Before trying any new cleaning agent, test a small quantity in a small area over a period of ten days. Never use any new product (even those recommended here) without first testing it.
2. Amway products are derived from coconut oil. Shaklee products *may* have a soybean base (the company refuses to divulge the source of its products). Since soybean is a more likely allergen, do not use Basic H to wash floors and other large surfaces, since greater exposure to a substance increases the possibility of sensitization. If you know you are already sensitive to soybean or coconut, then, of course, avoid products that contain them.
3. The following and similar substances should be stored outside the home in a *detached* storage place (not an attached garage or storeroom), even if they are in tightly sealed containers: paints, solvents, lacquers, turpentine, lighter fluid, charcoal fire-starters, glues, nail polish and nail-polish remover, odoriferous soaps and detergents, polishes of all types (shoe, metal, furniture, floor), mops and cloths used for cleaning purposes, chlorine bleaches, ammonia, and all volatile substances—and any entity suspected of being noxious, whether or not it has an objectionable odor.

Maintaining a healthy home doesn't end inside the house. The yard may also contribute to indoor pollution, particularly in the summer. First rule for the chemically sensitive person: Use no herbicides, insecticides, or fungicides. You may not have as good-looking a lawn as your neighbors who are using poisons, but a beautifully manicured lawn is a badge of pollution. The biocides that must be used to achieve a golf-course look evaporate and bathe your home in an invisible mist of chemicals that until recently never existed on the face of the earth. You can be certain that you will be breathing them to some extent even though you can't detect them. Some of the chemicals have already been cited as carcinogenic; long-term effects of the others are still unknown.

From a greater ecological point of view, water running off a beautiful lawn eventually finds its way into the groundwater, streams, and rivers, and eventually we'll all either be drinking it in our water supply or eating it in our fish.

One solution to the lawn problem is to use some sort of ground cover, such as crown vetch, a plant that needs practically no care, grows prolifically on its own, and has lovely purplish-pink flowers. Or consider a ground cover without plants such as crushed stone, rocks, and boulders, as used in Japanese gardens.[4]

The vegetable garden may also contribute to your household pollution. The mulch that is customarily used —hay, dried leaves, lawn clippings—produces prolific amounts of mold. If you live downwind from such a garden, your vegetables will be healthy, but you may not be. The solution here, of course, is to plant your garden downwind of the house. Or you can use a black plastic cover with vegetables planted in holes cut into it. The plastic acts as a "mulch," prevents weeds from growing, and retains water as well.[5]

All other things being equal, a homeowner might as well arrange his environment to be as compatible—as "natural," in most cases—as possible. And living in a chemically compatible environment is rarely more expensive, and indeed can often be cheaper, than surrounding oneself with toxins. You don't *have* to wax floors or polish furniture or spray for flies or even live in the most polluted section of your city. The catch phrase presented in Chapter 3 could well be repeated for emphasis here: If you can't eat it, don't breathe it.

PART III

Building the Healthy House

8

Selecting a Healthful Site

A hundred years ago, the place where one spent his life was pretty well predetermined; most people lived within perhaps a thirty-mile radius of where they were born. No longer; in today's mobile society few Americans live anywhere near their hometowns. At various times in the average person's life, he has a clear choice to make as to where he will live—in what section of the country, in what particular house—but among all the various factors to consider when selecting a place to live, most people give health barely a thought.

What were the considerations that went into the decision to live where *you* do? If you were not particularly environmentally aware, health was probably not one of them. And yet the health factor, the potential debilitating effects of pollution or allergens, may very well be *the* most important consideration. If you selected an environmentally detrimental location, it could affect you for the rest of your life, causing you to achieve less than your potential, producing a kind of sluggishness of thinking, a chronic touch of depression, a slow sapping of energy, a smothering, gentle fog of confusion. Perhaps nothing harmful would happen, but all other things being equal, why take a chance? If it has little effect on other considerations, one should select a house or apartment in a geographically healthful area, on a site that *adds* to the body's well-being.

Rule number one: If at all possible, get out of the city. The more congestion, the higher the pollution. Even if you don't smoke, if you live in a metropolitan area, you may be breathing the equivalent volume of some of those same carcinogenic chemicals anyway. For example, one of the substances in tobacco smoke blamed for lung cancer is the hydrocarbon benzpyrene. A person smoking one pack of cigarettes a day might be exposing himself to sixty micrograms of benzpyrene over a year. If he didn't smoke, and lived in the mountains of, say, Montana, he might inhale only one-tenth of one microgram in the same time. Yet a U.S. Public Health Service pamphlet estimates that "the average quantities of benzpyrene inhaled by persons exposed [to] the air of some cities over a year's time might equal as much benzpyrene as from smoking two packs of cigarettes daily."[1] Another statistic: One milliliter of air in the wilderness contains an average of about 6,000 particles; in cities, the count zooms to several *million*.

Cities are detrimental electrically too. On the one hand, microwave and other high-frequency radiation usually saturates urban areas. And on the other, the ion count in cities is almost always low, mainly because of the air pollution.[2] An estimated 60 percent of the population of North America spends about 80 percent of its time in cities and urban areas, where the total ion count is hopelessly depleted, electromagnetic radiation is awesome in its quantity, and general pollution is staggering.

If you *must* live in a city or its environs, however, note that some neighborhoods are better than others. In fact, it might be a good idea to plot major pollution sources on a map before you begin house hunting. The prevailing winds over most of the United States come from the west or northwest, so start your search for a house or apartment on the western side of town—*far* to the west of such major pollution sources as factories, industrial parks, large highways, and railroads. Avoid, too, locations next to large parking lots; choose a residence there and you'll be suffocated not only in exhaust fumes, but if the surface is tarred or asphalted, in petrochemical vapors as well. Airports should be especially avoided. A modern jet liner upon takeoff produces the pollution equivalent of nearly seven thousand automobiles.[3] And homes within a mile or more may be bathed in the airport's radar system. (You'll also be subjected to noise, another form of pollution.)

The lot itself should be as large as you can afford, with the house in the center, surrounded by a buffer zone between yourself and the outside world. If your city is hilly, look for a house on one of the crests; valleys tend to have relatively stagnant air, pollution-rich, and with diminished ion concentrations as well.[4] (Air ion concentration increases with height.) A hillside house can be basking in sunshine and clean air, while people in the valley below cough and grope their way through the day. (Your garden, too, will do better up there, and if you have your own well, it is less susceptible to groundwater contamination.) It's the same thing with an apartment; the higher the floor, the fewer fumes will likely breeze in your window. Apartments on lower floors are assaulted not only by street pollution but often by gases from connected garages as well. (Some building designs, in fact, allow fumes from basement garages and furnace rooms to flow up elevator shafts to befoul upper hallways.[5]) High-level apartments may present one danger, however. If a television transmitter is near (some cities place such towers on the taller buildings), the upper apartments might be bathed in radiation at severely high levels. The Office of Telecommunications Policy *Annual Report* for 1973 stated that "levels of two milliwatts per square centimeter or higher in nearby high structures" may exist near TV transmitters—an amount that's not unlawful but is medically highly questionable.

Some cities are considerably worse than others. Portland, Oregon, was cited in a 1978 Environmental Protection Agency report as having the highest concentration of microwaves of twelve metropolitan areas studied. Chicago human ecologist Theron Randolph cites the following areas as some of "the very worst, polluted places to stay away from":

1. East Chicago, Gary, Whiting, and Hammond areas. Even people who are driving through the state, says Randolph, should detour around this area, or "close their windows on Calumet Skyway and leave them closed until arriving on the other side of Gary." One study revealed that in Chicago, residential and industrial chimneys produce enough particulate matter that an average of thirty-seven tons a year settles down on every square mile within the city limits.

2. The Sarnia area of Canada, south of Lake Huron, the refinery center of Canada.

3. East of El Paso, Texas, with its many oil refineries.

4. The entire Gulf Coast area from New Orleans to Padre Island, because of numerous refineries and chemical-manufacturing plants.

5. The Imperial Valley in California and the artichoke area near Salinas, California, which is heavily sprayed with pesticides.

6. The Kanawha Valley and Charleston, West Virginia, and the Pittsburgh-Wheeling area to central Ohio, because of industrial smog.

7. Perth Amboy, New Jersey, south of New York City, and east of New Brunswick, also because of its industrial pollution. "The area is unfit for human habitation," says Randolph.[6]

In fact, all of northeastern New Jersey is questionable. With more than 7 million people squeezed into only 7,521 square miles, New Jersey is the most densely populated state in the nation—and one of the most industrialized as well. It once dubbed itself "The Nation's Chemical Capital." Now others are giving it another designation: "The Nation's Cancer Capital." A 1975 publication released by the National Cancer Institute put all twenty-one of New Jersey's counties in the top 10 percent for overall cancer mortality.[7] New Jersey's mortality rate for urinary and bladder cancer, closely associated with exposure to industrial chemicals, is half again as high as for the nation as a whole. At least seven potential carcinogens have been detected in New Jersey air, and in March 1978, when 250 wells were tested in twelve New Jersey counties, nearly all of them were found to contain trace amounts of foreign chemicals, including such likely cancer causers as carbon tetrachloride, vinyl chloride, and a variety of pesticides.

Randolph also cites three environmentally beneficial places to live: Oregon or Washington; central Kansas, Nebraska, and eastern Montana; and the southern Appalachians (even though some sensitive people find the pollen count there excessive).

A factor that isn't so directly related to health, but to comfort, is climate—and it can vary enormously within only a few hundred feet, horizontally or vertically. In California, the temperature may be 60 degrees near the ocean and 105 degrees just a few miles eastward on the other side of the coastal ridges. Some parts of Hawaii receive more than 200 inches of rainfall a year, other parts less than 15. And many areas of the country are subjected to bitterly cold winds, while a few miles to either side, calm or gentle eddies prevail. If you are moving to a mountainous area especially, it would be wise to visit the local weather bureau for guidance. And while you're there, look at the records of hailstorms, heavy snows, hurricanes, and tornadoes too.

When you look for a residence, you'll also want to keep an eye out for transmission lines, broadcast towers, and microwave-relay stations. A house that's too close should be rejected. How close? Nobody knows for sure. Although living next to a broadcasting tower or between microwave-relay stations or adjacent to transmission lines has been shown to have an adverse effect on human beings, the specific distance at which this effect becomes insignificant is still a point of considerable controversy. The only thing that can be said with certainty: the farther the better. Perhaps a rough yardstick is that if, from your prospective site, you can *see* the towers from ground level, search out another location.

If you are one of the 35 million Americans (estimated by the American Academy of Allergy) who are sensitive to pollen, you may want to head toward a relatively pollen-free area. Ragweed, probably the pollen that causes the most misery among Americans, can be largely escaped by moving to the desert regions and forests of the Rockies; the southern tip of Florida and the Florida Keys (because they're surrounded by water); the forest areas of New Hampshire, northern Maine, and extreme northern Michigan; and the whole West Coast, particularly west of the Cascade Mountains in Oregon and Washington. Or nearly anywhere other than North America. Ragweed grows in almost no other part of the world, including Hawaii and the Caribbean islands.

The heaviest ragweed concentration occurs in the Midwest, from about west-central South Dakota to Ohio, northern Pennsylvania, and central New York. Most of the East Coast has a substantial ragweed density, as does western Texas and eastern Montana. The Plains states and the mountain states are relatively free of ragweed. However, ragweed-sensitive individuals usually develop sagebrush allergy in these areas. In northeastern Colorado and western Nebraska, tumbleweed pollen causes problems. In Utah and Wyoming, add the Mexican firebush.

Unfortunately, even a highly allergic person can't rely on his own symptoms to tell him when he's in a pollen-safe area. Everyone requires a period of sensitization before he reacts to a new allergen. If you're from Connecticut, for example, and visit Oregon for the first time, you probably can live there for a number of months or years allergy-free, or you may *never* develop a new sensitivity. Or you may be sneezing next summer. There's just no way to predict.

So to be safe, you'll have to move to a region with very little, not simply *different*, pollen. Unfortunately, it's not so easy to escape pollen as it used to be. Twenty years ago, Marcia Newman, a writer who suffers from asthma, moved from Pennsylvania to Tucson to escape ragweed pollen. "It was the best move I ever made," she told me not long ago. "The air was dry, it was clean, it was free of pollen, and I forgot what it was to wheeze." In the last few years, though, she's relearned what it was like. Two decades ago, Tucson's population stood at a little over 45,000. Now it's nearly six times that, and Ms. Newman, now sixty-two, is wheezing, sneezing, and coughing just as in the bad old days. What has happened to the air in the meantime? The newcomers brought with them not only general pollution but Eastern tastes for thick hedges and extensive gardens, and now, according to *Time,* in a kind of pollen pollution, dust from thousands of mulberry shade trees and other nonnative flora floats cloudlike through the dry air—unlike pollen from most of Arizona's native plants, which relies on birds and insects to pass from flower to flower.[8] What's even worse, Tucson's growing season lasts most of the year. Some of the imported plants produce pollen from February to October, and the dry wind can blow it for hundreds of miles.

You could of course be certain of pollen-free air by moving in with the two dozen researchers at Byrd Station, South Pole. But if you don't want to go that far, the best place is either to the oceanside, in an area where sea breezes blow inland constantly, or high in the mountains. The mountains, in fact, with their heavier concentration of ions and relatively pollution-free atmosphere, make the best all-around choice for a homesite.

And that isn't just theory. In 1977, a team of researchers from Harvard, Case Western Reserve, and the University of New Mexico released an extensive, thirteen-year study of people living in high altitudes of New Mexico. They discovered little of significance concerning women. But for men the death rate from coronary heart disease was 28 percent lower among those who lived above 7,000 feet than among those who lived at 3,000 to 4,000 feet.[9]

One other important consideration in selecting a new home or homesite is the water supply. Few people know exactly where their municipal drinking water comes from, and fewer still care. Most Americans believe that toxins—pesticides, industrial runoff, herbicides, animal-feed hormones, human intestinal viruses—have been removed from their drinking water before it reaches their taps. Such is not the case. In 1970 a coast-to-coast survey by the federal Bureau of Water Hygiene, the largest such sampling ever conducted in this country, revealed the astonishing fact that nearly a third of the water samples taken in homes contained chemicals in quantities exceeding the limits recommended by the U.S. Public Health Service.[10] Nine out of ten municipal water-treatment systems in the United States were designed to kill bacteria and to strain out the larger chunks of matter, but *not* to remove toxic chemicals, or even all viruses. As a result, millions of Americans are drinking contaminated water, essentially recycled sewage and industrial waste drawn from such poisoned waterways as Lake Erie, Lake Michigan, the Potomac, Mississippi, and Hudson rivers, and dozens of lesser-known streams and lakes. As quoted in a 1971 Ralph Nader study group report, James McDermott, then director of the Bureau of Water Hygiene, said that "aside from occasional irritation associated with taste and odor problems, overconfidence or apathy seems to pervade the public's attitude with respect to drinking water."[11] And the Nader group adds this comment: "Many state health officials seem to have become security-conscious administrators who believe that maintaining public trust is at least as important as protecting the water itself."[12]

Two adjacent towns may have entirely different sources of water—one heavily infused with exotic chemicals, the other free of contaminants. For example, along the banks of the Hudson River as it flows from Albany to New York City, scores of cities and towns sprawl elbow to elbow. Some use the river as a water supply. Some don't. Nearly all of them dump their "treated" sewage into the river, mixing it with the outflow of the 254 industries permitted to discharge pollutants (and all the others who aren't, but do anyway). In September 1977 a report compiled by the Environmental Defense Fund and the New York Public Interest Research Group stated that "the lives of 150,000 people who drink water from the

Hudson may be in danger because existing filtration systems can't screen out . . . toxic chemicals." It cited some of the chemicals now being poured into the Hudson: benzene, tetrahydrofuran, polychlorinated biphenyls (PCB), cyclohexane, methylbenz(a)anthracene, toluene, dibutyphthalate, xylene—all labeled "hazardous."[13]

The fact is, though, the Hudson is not all that outstanding. For its size and use, it's one of America's cleaner rivers. And yet at least 150,000 people are drinking potentially hazardous chemicals, while hundreds of thousands more along its banks live in communities that get their water from clear mountain streams carefully administered to prevent pollution. Conclusion: When you are shopping around for a homesite, check the source of the municipal water. A shift in location of only a few miles may make the difference between water that's heavily contaminated and water that's pollution-free.

Not so easy to get away from is chlorine. The fact that chlorine is a potential threat should not be a surprise; as far back as 1934 *The Journal of Allergy* carried an article by two Tucson physicians that cited chlorinated water as a cause of asthma.[14] For the chlorine-sensitive person, a shower with chlorine-treated water can trigger all manner of problems, because the heating and splashing of the water aerosolizes chlorene-infused droplets and liberates quantities of gas, both to be breathed in the confines of the shower stall. The dissolved gas is also released when heated—in the laundry, for example, or in a swimming pool, or even in a closed bathroom from a hot tub of water. It all becomes part of the house's general atmosphere.

For those who are not obviously sensitive to chlorine, what is the long-term effect of drinking the gas? It is after all, a virulent poison; that's why it kills bacteria so effectively. The answer: Nobody knows.

What *is* known, however, is that a startling correlation exists between chlorinated water and certain types of cancer. From 1966 to 1970 Dr. Michael Alvanja, an assistant professor in environmental health and epidemiology at Hunter College in New York City, in a program funded by the government's Environmental Protection Agency, studied records of 1,595 women who died from urinary-tract or gastrointestinal cancer in seven New York counties. When he compared the water in the homes of those women, he made an alarming discovery: Those who drank chlorinated water ran a 44 percent higher chance of dying from the cancers than those who drank untreated water.

One possible explanation is that when chlorine interacts with dissolved organic material it produces multiple types of chlorinated hydrocarbons, including chloroform, a known carcinogen. The Environmental Protection Agency, suggesting that the chloroform limit be placed at 100 parts per billion (a figure that some feel is too high), released the accompanying table of eighty U.S. cities and their chloroform levels.

There *are* alternatives to using chlorine, by the way. One popular method used in the Soviet Union and some 200 European cities is ozone treatment. Ozone is so unstable that by the time the water reaches the house, the gas has disappeared, having decomposed into oxygen. Another method is to pass water to be treated through microwaves. Both systems kill bacteria as effectively as does chlorine. A combination of ultrasound and ozone (called *sonocatalytic ozonation*) cuts the cost by half, making it competitive with chlorination.[15] But so far, no alternative to chlorine has sparked much interest in this country. To my knowledge, the only U.S. community to use ozone treatment for its drinking water is Whiting, Indiana.[16]

To rid water of chlorine in your home, boil it for two or three minutes, or let it stand overnight. You'll be breathing some of the gas, but you won't ingest it in such concentrated quantities.

Another method to rid the water of chlorine (and certain other impurities, including chloroform) is to install a charcoal filter on the water tap. But I don't recommend it. Such filters probably create more problems than they solve. In a series of tests run by the Department of Virology and Epidemiology of Houston's Baylor College of

Medicine, researchers found that under typical home conditions, bacteria populations within a week multiplied some 70,000 times. One company, in an attempt to eliminate this hazard, impregnates its carbon filters with silver. But when the Department of Environmental and Community Services in Idaho measured the silver leached out, it found it to be at levels several times that which the Public Health Service had recommended as "maximum permissible." (Ingested silver can cause lifetime discoloration of the mucous membranes, eyes, and skin.)

Even if the water enters your home pristine-pure, your house itself may contribute to its pollution. If your home is very old and your lead pipes have never been replaced, tiny amounts of lead might be leaching out of them, and even doses below toxic levels can contribute to poor health.[17] Galvanized pipe, too, can be a source of health problems. It's not the zinc coating that causes the trouble, but the trace amounts of cadmium that some galvanizing processes include. As water courses through the pipes, it may pick up small amounts of cadmium, which, in turn—because its chemical activity is similar to zinc—displaces zinc in the body. Cadmium has been implicated as a possible cause of hypertension,[18] and what's more, it inhibits the immune system, the system responsible for, among other things, fighting off infection and destroying cancer cells.[19] Even polyvinylchloride plastic pipe may impart cadmium to the water supply, because cadmium is used in the plasticizer.[20] The best selection is copper pipe with flare fittings (further discussed in Chapter 9).

One means of protecting against the onslaught of cadmium is to increase the dietary intake of zinc. (Dietary zinc supplement is available in many health-food stores as zinc sulfate, zinc citrate, or zinc glucolate. Recommended dose: 15 milligrams twice a week together with a good diet.) Another is to live in an area in which the water happens to have a high selenium content. Selenium seems somehow to counteract cadmium's effects.[21]

One thing you *don't* have to worry about is hard water. Welcome it. There's solid statistical evidence that

CHLOROFORM—

	PARTS PER BILLION		PARTS PER BILLION
ALASKA		**KANSAS**	
Douglas	40	Topeka	88
ARIZONA		**KENTUCKY**	
Phoenix	9	Owensboro	13
Tucson	0.2	**LOUISIANA**	
ARKANSAS		Houma	134
Camden	40	Logansport	28
CALIFORNIA		**MARYLAND**	
Coalinga	16	Baltimore	32
Cobcord	31	**MASSACHUSETTS**	
Dos Palos	61	Boston	4
Los Angeles	32	Lawrence	91
San Diego	52	**MICHIGAN**	
San Francisco	41	Detroit	12
COLORADO		Mt. Clemens	11
Denver	14	**MINNESOTA**	
Pueblo	2	St. Paul	44
CONNECTICUT		**MISSISSIPPI**	
Waterbury	93	Greenville	17
DELAWARE		**MISSOURI**	
Claymont	23	Kansas City	24
Newark	0.5	St. Louis	55
DISTRICT OF COLUMBIA	41	**NEBRASKA**	
FLORIDA		Lincoln	4
Jacksonville	9	**NEW JERSEY**	
Miami	311	Little Falls	59
GEORGIA		Toms River	0.6
Atlanta	36	**NEW MEXICO**	
IDAHO		Albuquerque	0.4
Idaho Falls	2	**NEW YORK**	
ILLINOIS		Buffalo	10
Chicago	15	New York City	22
Clinton	4	Rhinebeck	49
INDIANA		**NORTH DAKOTA**	
Indianapolis	31	Grand Forks	3
Whiting	0.5	**OHIO**	
IOWA		Cincinnati	45
Clarinda	48	Cleveland	18
Davenport	88	Columbus	134
Ottumwa	0.8	Dayton	8

Indian Hill	5	Memphis	0.9
Picqua	131	Nashville	16
Youngstown	80	TEXAS	
OKLAHOMA		Brownsville	12
Oklahoma City	44	Dallas	18
OREGON		San Antonio	0.2
Corvallis	26	UTAH	
PENNSYLVANIA		Salt Lake City	20
Philadelphia	86	VIRGINIA	
Pittsburgh	8	Annandale	67
Strasburg	0.1	Hopewell	6
PUERTO RICO		WASHINGTON	
San Juan	47	Ilwaco	167
RHODE ISLAND		Seattle	15
Newport	103	WEST VIRGINIA	
SOUTH CAROLINA		Huntington	23
Charleston	195	Wheeling	72
SOUTH DAKOTA		WISCONSIN	
Huron	309	Milwaukee	9
TENNESSEE		Oshkosh	26
Chattanooga	30		

States where no testing was done: Alabama, Hawaii, Maine, Montana, Nevada, New Hampshire, North Carolina, Vermont, Wyoming.

For the chloroform level in your town, call the local water company. (Odd that one should telephone for the "accepted poison level.")

---

people who drink hard water (from such natural, dissolved substances as calcium, magnesium, sulfate, and bicarbonate) tend to have a smaller incidence of high blood pressure and cardiovascular problems than those who live in soft-water areas. This remarkable discovery came about after the U.S. Geological Survey tested municipal water in 1,315 American cities, representing 90 percent of the country's urban population. The water was checked for hardness, and the figures were correlated with death rates from cardiovascular disease. The fact clearly emerged that if one drinks hard instead of soft water, he is less likely to have a heart attack. Therefore, it's better *not* to install a water-softening unit in the home unless on a system separate from the drinking water. Furthermore, artificially softened water is laden with excessive salts, a potential contributing factor in elevated blood pressure.

Exactly why hard water seems to be beneficial remains obscure, but one hypothesis comes from Dr. Henry A. Schroeder, the physician who conducted the original study. He presents as "a modicum of speculation" the idea that soft waters in particular "attack the pipes through which they run, taking up zinc, cadmium, iron, copper or lead, depending on the kind of pipes and solders used. In that event, cadmium or lead might be suspect; both accumulate in human tissues."[22] And cadmium uptake has long been identified as one cause of high blood pressure and coronary heart disease.

The danger from drinking chlorinated water, or soft water, and even of inadequately recycled sewage and industrial wastes, is, in the whole order of things, relatively small. At least it is not an immediate cause of certain death. But again, all other things being equal, you might as well select a town with a water source that doesn't need heavy treatment. Or dig your own well.

Not everyone can live just where he wants to, of course. The specialist in elevator repairing can't take his trade to the Ozarks, nor can the steelworker easily quit and move to a Caribbean island. Within reason, though, nearly everyone has *some* choice—this apartment or that, this neighborhood or that. And the primary factor that should go into the formula to determine where to live is health.

Designing the Healthy House

A physician keeps current by reading scientific literature, by attending conferences, and by taking advanced courses in his specialty. His *real* education, however, comes from his patients: He not only advises them, he learns from them. The polite greeting "How are you?" is used by everyone, but the physician listens to the answers, and each response goes into his computer-bank mind as another modicum of data, another bit of evidence. Over the years, my patients have been teaching me a great deal, and they keep me informed; they let me know when ragweed season begins, when the mold count is high, which geographic areas are healthy and which are not. They've taught me that painting in winter is detrimental, that household "deodorizers" are harmful, that cooking with gas can be hazardous.

So when I decided to build a new house, I applied the accumulated experiences of my environmentally sensitive patients to the plans, using their case histories to guide me in the selection of many of the components. Frank Lloyd Wright once said that he could design a house that would ensure that the occupants would get divorced. And I could design one that would make the householders sick.

As an ecologically oriented physician, I was guided by

my patients almost as though they were biological essays. For example, through clinical observation, I verified the theory of the best place to live; I found that in my particular county, when my sensitive patients visit an area some two dozen miles northwest of Kingston, New York, in the higher elevations of the Catskills, they benefit. And I saw that if patients who had been living in those higher elevations moved into one of the towns lining the Hudson (with the resulting increase in pollution and decrease in ions), they suffered.

I realized that since I was going to build a house, I should take advantage of the opportunity to do it right, to design one that would not only enhance my family's health but would serve as a model for future medical observation. And I realized that if my house turned out to be less healthful than it might have been, it would not be the fault of the architect or professional builder; it would be mine, because although the building skills would come from others, the medical judgments would come from me.

What finally resulted, after years of study and design, is, to my knowledge, the first domestic residence ever to be constructed with an orientation toward cellular physiology—the ultimate "form follows function."

In this chapter I'll show my steps, the thinking that went into the decisions, the selection of materials, the compromises. And if you build your own healthy house, you might want to follow some of the same procedures.

First, placement is all-important. Because of the prevailing winds, I selected a site far to the west of the Hudson Valley industry, west of major highways, and far from high-tension lines, microwave-relay towers, and broadcasting stations. I aimed for a high elevation—2,200 feet above sea level—wanting to get away from valley pollution, to benefit from increased ion density, and to capture summer breezes.

After selecting the site, I went through the same kind of self-analysis every home builder does when he chooses a design: I had to find out just who I am, and what I and my family want and need in a house. No architect can interpret the owner's needs better than the client himself. Besides, as Ken Kern points out in *The Owner-Built Home*, "Most contemporary architects design houses for themselves, not their clients. They work at satisfying some esthetic whim, and fail really to understand the character of the site and the personal requirements of the client."[1] And of course, the word "health" has not yet entered the ordinary architect's vocabulary. It took me two years to find an architect and an engineer who would be receptive to a physiological approach to building.

When I decided what my family and I wanted—the number of rooms, kinds of rooms, activity centers, flow —I called in the architect and the engineer to fill in the details. We worked closely in the selection of materials, discussing every detail in depth, taking into consideration practicality, cost, aesthetics, availability of materials, difficulty of construction, and, above all, health.

One thing that I discovered through these discussions is that building a healthy house is no more expensive than constructing a conventional dwelling. Individual components may cost more (the initial outlay for a heat pump is higher than for an oil-fired furnace, for instance), but in other areas, one saves. The elimination of a basement, for example, can cut costs by thousands of dollars. So when all the expenses are added up, the figures show that one can build a house that promotes either health or illness for about the same cost.

Speaking of basements, that was one of the first things to be cut from the design. Rex Roberts, in *Your Engineered House*, goes on at some length about basements. Says he (in part):

> Why anyone, nowadays, should dig a big hole in the ground and then put a house in it escapes me completely. . . . The historical and technical reasons for basements have long since disappeared. There is not one single thing on my list of day-round and year-round activities that I would put in a basement unless the basement were already there. . . . Once the potato bin, coal bin, and jam shelves have quit

working, it's better to fix up a basement for something else than to let the rats move in. But it's expensive. . . .

Only with effort and expense can a basement be kept anywhere near as warm, dry, light, quiet, clean, useful and pleasant as the same amount of space on a ground floor can be for less money. . . . I'm stumped. The emotional need to get onto an upper floor I can understand, but when it comes to basements, I can't even think of an emotional reason.[2]

I agree. And Roberts wasn't even considering health. Look at the basement through the eyes of a physician, and the mold problem alone is enough to eliminate it from your plans.

What would you put in a basement? Washing machine? Workshop? Furnace? The laundry room can go on the first floor, where circulating air carries off the moisture, the chlorine fumes, the vapors from cleaning agents. And it's handier there too, and has a more pleasant atmosphere. The workshop can also go on the main floor—or better, in another building, so that sawdust and paint fumes and other noxious vapors won't drift into the living quarters. In my case, I've built a separate structure. It holds a workshop, a small laboratory, and my garage.

I especially wanted the garage to be in a detached structure. *Attached* garages flood the home with exhaust fumes and vapors from evaporating oil and gasoline every time the connecting door is opened. An attached garage is further unacceptable because the wall cannot be made vaporproof. I found it just as easy to design a separate structure connected to the house by a covered walkway open to the breeze.

If I had decided to install an oil-fired furnace, that would have gone in that detached building too. A furnace room *can* be attached to the main house, but it must be sealed off, accessible only from the outside, with an outside source of combustion. One terrible location for a furnace is where it's most often placed: under the main section of the house. But if placed well away from the living quarters (and downwind as well) and if the only direct connections to the home are the water lines, even a fossil-fuel furnace is acceptable. The main consideration here is the possibility of an oil leak, and the question: If oil is spilled, would the furnace-room location allow oil vapors to contaminate the house?

Steam heat, by the way, is rarely used today, and because most steam systems are of the *gravity* type, the furnace must be in the basement—unacceptable in the healthy house. In addition, steam systems release chlorine into the room air, inducing chronic symptoms in certain sensitive persons.

A gas- or oil-fueled furnace is *not* recommended, even in a detached building, if a forced-air system is used; the possibilities of a break in the firebox are too great. And there is no easy way of monitoring (or even testing) a system to see that the firebox is still intact, although a few quite expensive, permanently installed gas-detection units are available that will sound a warning signal or shut down the furnace.

Resistance-wire electric heat is very good; it eliminates the furnace completely and is relatively inexpensive to buy and to install. But it has a number of drawbacks: (1) Straight resistance is the most expensive heat source to operate, and it is likely to become more so in the fuel-lean years ahead. (2) It has no built-in mechanism for humidity control. (3) Still somewhat controversial is the "fried dust" phenomenon, the heating of dust as it passes over hot resistance coils, which is suspected of enhancing its allergenic potential. (4) Particles of plastic (from carpets, for instance) heated by the coils may depolymerize—break down into simpler molecules—and release toxic fumes. (5) Finally, heating elements that reach the temperature required in *central* electric systems may produce positive ions, upsetting the home's electrical atmosphere.

The best all-around system, and the one installed in my home, is a heat pump, widely used in the South but only recently with advanced technology becoming established in northern states. This is a device that extracts heat from the air at one point and deposits it at another.

A refrigerator is a heat pump; it sucks heat from the inside air and moves it into the kitchen. A window air conditioner is a heat pump too, pulling heat from the room and releasing it outside. A total-house heat pump, connected to a ductwork system, acts much like a conventional air-conditioning system in the summer, and, reversed, as a furnace in the winter. Surprisingly, no matter how cold the winter air becomes, it still contains a great deal of heat, and this can be extracted and moved into the home, while air returned to the outside is even cooler than when it came in. Most units include a supplementary resistance-heating system that automatically begins operating when the temperature drops below freezing. The initial cost is somewhat above that of a conventional furnace, and the operating cost (at this writing) is still more than for oil or gas in the North, because electric heat must be used during cold weather when heat pumps cannot supply enough heat for comfort. Nevertheless, operating costs for heat pumps are less than that for straight-resistance heat. And as fuel prices inflate, heat-pump operating expenses will become competitive with oil and gas. Another big advantage of the heat pump is that it operates at a lower temperature than resistance heating—about 90 degrees F.—and so is less likely to develop the "fried dust" phenomenon or to depolymerize plastic particles.

If you have a fairly good groundwater supply (three gallons a minute or so), you might consider a *water-source* heat pump, one that extracts heat from a backyard well. The advantage of this system is that groundwater is always the average annual temperature of the ambient air—always above freezing (unless you live in a permafrost region)—so even in subzero temperatures, no straight-resistance heating is necessary. As of this writing, the Vaughn Corporation produces the best unit for northern climates, while any number of manufacturers make water-source heat pumps suitable for heating and cooling in southern weather.[3]

As solar-heating technology becomes refined and commercially more feasible, solar systems should also be considered, either alone or in conjunction with a heat pump.[4] As with other systems, humidification and filtration devices must be integrated. Theoretically, from a health standpoint, solar systems should be superior to conventional units, mainly because of the absence of fuel vapors. One possible source of trouble, however, is in a solar system's heat sink, the area where daytime heat is stored for nighttime release. Some systems use a huge vat of water for heat storage, and this should cause no problem. But other designs call for a large quantity of stones or other material, and this kind of sink may be a source of mold and other particle contaminants. As of this writing, however, so few solar systems have been installed that no health evidence has surfaced.

In any home heating system, more is involved than simply warming the air. Some method of controlling humidity must be installed, along with a means for air filtration. The only system that can effectively deal with all three factors is a network of ducts. Some physicians feel that a hot-air system is undesirable, and they give two main reasons: It tends to blow dust around, and it eliminates negative ions. It *does* blow dust around, but only if the home is quite dusty to begin with and the filtering system is inadequate. I find that if a home is properly maintained and if the filters are regularly changed, a house served by forced air is considerably cleaner than one heated by another system, mainly because it is constantly cleaning itself by forcing air through filters. The negative-ion problem is a real one, but I feel that the advantages of an air system outweigh that objection.

Maintaining proper humidity is of vital importance. It affects our health and comfort, and lowers the heating bill as well. During the colder winter weather, the relative humidity, a measure of the ability of the air to absorb moisture, drops drastically. Cold outside air, because it *is* cold, simply cannot hold much moisture, and so the *total* amount of water vapor is very low. When the air enters the home (and there is always some inside/outside circulation), it is heated to a comfortable temperature, which increases its ability to hold a larger quantity of water vapor. Because the percentage of saturation (the relative humidity) of the outside air is low, and the air quite dry, the evaporation of any available water inside the home is rapid. The air acts like a sponge, gathering moisture from wherever it can. That's why dampness—in the kitchen, basement, or bath—is less of a problem in winter; the air is absorbing it all.

That's fine, but at less than a comfortable 30 to 40 percent or so, the air also has a severe drying effect on the protective linings of the nose, throat, and lungs—and many medical researchers now believe that this is a major reason people have more colds during the winter months. Dry nasal linings can't function so effectively, and their ability to combat viruses is impaired. So we come down with colds. In addition, dry air holds fewer ions—and that, too, might be a reason for so many winter colds.

A common method for humidifying a home is to install a central humidifier in the air-circulating system. Such a device does the job if the humidifier is attached to the ductwork at an appropriate place for easy maintenance. Some manufacturers of humidifiers, anticipating a mold problem, recommend the addition of Clorox or other toxins—a practice that shouldn't even be considered; the chemicals aerosolize into the air, to be breathed by everyone in the household.

One alternative to the central system is a portable humidifier with a plastic tank easily removed for cleaning. (Scrub with a stiff vegetable brush under running water, without soap, once a week.) The fact that the humidifier isn't connected to the central system makes little difference in vapor distribution. Humidity will eventually float more or less evenly throughout the house in either case; it simply is distributed faster with a forced-air system.

The other alternative to a duct system is a built-in unit—often in a closet, with the moisture breezing into the room through a hole in the wall. One big problem with some such units, however, is that they inject aerosolized water *particles* into the air rather than water *vapor*. The disadvantage here is that any dissolved minerals or suspended mold, bacteria, or algae that happen to be in the water will remain in the droplets, floating through the house to be breathed by the occupants, with a real danger of disease or allergy as a result. The minerals eventually settle out as a powdery deposit on all nearby surfaces.

Other built-in models, though, rely not on water injection, but strictly on evaporation—and when water evaporates, it leaves the minerals and other matter behind. With these units, air is blown over a reservoir electrically heated, resulting in "enhanced" evaporation.

One particularly efficient humidifier of the built-in, enhanced-evaporation type, made by Humid-Aire (model 315 or MA-115), is connected directly to a water supply, which eliminates the nuisance of filling the tank by hand. And it's wired to the duct-system blower so that maximum evaporation occurs only when the air is being circulated.

Incidentally, contrary to what one might expect, such a heated unit is energy-efficient. A gram of water requires 540 calories of heat to evaporate. In a conventional system the heat comes from the reservoir water, and the water cools; it is reheated by the room air, which ultimately is warmed by the home heating system. (In most climates the humidifier will be running only during the winter.) An internally warmed unit does draw current, but the cost, strange as it might seem, works out to be identical with a nonheated model.

A humidifier has another advantage too: A house of high humidity *feels* warmer. The dryer the air, the faster perspiration evaporates, and the skin too loses 540 calories of heat for each gram of perspiration that changes to a gas. In a humid atmosphere, perspiration evaporates slowly, and so the skin actually *is* warmer, and you can set your thermostat back a bit. A humidifier, then—conventional or internally heated—actually cuts the total energy bill.

Another important effect of low humidity is electrical. High humidity allows electricity to flow through the air to the ground. But in dry, winter air, when you walk across a carpet, you build up a charge in your body, released as a "static-electric" spark when you touch a conductor. This never happens in the summer. In an atmosphere made more humid by a humidifier, the charge tends to leak off into the air.

In summer, of course, you have the opposite problem: excessive humidity. When high temperatures combine with high humidity, perspiration fails to evaporate quickly, and discomfort results. A 72-degree day in Houston with a relative humidity of 90 percent and barely moving air will give an *effective* temperature of 80 degrees F. In Albuquerque, with the relative humidity at 10 percent, the wind about one mph, and the temperature at a blistering 100 degrees F., the effective temperature is still only 80 degrees F., because perspiration evaporates quickly. The point here is that an air-conditioning system must remove moisture as well as cool the air, or the occupant of the home will feel clammy.

To check the humidity in your present home, you can use what is called a sling psychrometer (also a dry-bulb/wet-bulb hygrometer), sold in heating and plumbing supply stores. It's composed of two thermometers, one with a wick wrapped around the bulb. When dipped in water and whirled into the air, the double thermometer produces two temperatures that, when compared (as detailed on the instruction sheet supplied with the unit), indicate the relative humidity.

A further word about air conditioning: Most ecologists and others interested in saving energy disdain it. They feel that it is unnecessary, that proper design of a home to capture prevailing breezes—to allow air to sweep through, flushing the hot, inside air up and out vents near the top of the house—makes it a foolish luxury. I agree, and excellent information is available on designing homes so that natural ventilation will do a satisfactory summer cooling job.[5] For example, most homes provide for attic ventilation by the installation of louvered vents at each end of the attic. A more efficient system is a "continuous ridge vent" combined with eave vents (see Appendix B).

For the hay-fever sufferer, however, over much of the U.S. climate, *only* properly filtered, forced-air ventilation will do the filtering and cooling job needed. Natural air circulation requires a free flow, and the filtering system necessary to rid the household air of pollen simply interferes too much with such a flow. A compromise for cooling (without filtration) is a simple fan system that would pull the air in at a low level, blowing it out the attic. I suggest that the house builder keep all systems in mind, that he design for natural ventilation, but that in times of heavy pollen concentration (unfortunately, usually directly proportional to the temperature), he have a forced-air cooling system available. Some days it might be enough to use ductwork and fans alone. But if you're going to install a duct system anyway—and particularly if you decide on a heat pump—you might as well install the *capacity* of a cooling system too.

The ductwork itself needs a close look. Built-in plastic dampers or air directors should not be used; the heat of the system in winter can contribute to slow depolymerization of the plastic, and the subsequent vapors may contribute to the general air pollution. Insulation should never be placed *within* a duct, only on the outside. Some heating contractors place material inside ducts to diminish noise, but this is dangerous: Passage of air will dislodge particles, and if the "soundproofing" materials are plastic, outgassing will likely result. One other thing: When the workmen are installing the ductwork, check to see that no oil is used to slide the sections together, or to protectively coat the metal. The residue, especially when heated, could evaporate and blow throughout the house. It eventually will be eliminated, but in the meantime you'll be breathing it.

At the time the ductwork was being planned for my house, I hired a firm specializing in built-in vacuuming systems. Installation and layout is best done by a company specializing in such work, not by a general or electrical contractor. The cost is the same, or even lower, and you will have a superior system. No matter who does the work, though, make sure that the exhaust outlet is *down-*

wind, and that the vacuum motor is installed at a site that is easily accessible for cleaning yet doesn't contribute to the household noise.

While the vacuuming system was being laid out, I planned the plumbing, and that took considerable thought. First, I rejected galvanized iron, not necessarily on health grounds (although the ingestion of small amounts of cadmium over the years is questionable), but for economy. The pipe itself is inexpensive, but installation labor isn't; and because iron pipe eventually rusts through, it rarely is installed in new homes today.

So the choice was between copper and plastic, and I selected copper. No direct evidence exists that plastic pipe imparts any more harmful chemicals to drinking water than copper, but virtually no studies have been done, and no long-term empirical data have been gathered. And because plastic is not really inert—it depolymerizes to some extent, becomes brittle over the years, and changes its chemistry—I felt that it would be wise to avoid it.

Flare fittings instead of solder joints were used in two runs: from the well to the main house supply, and from the supply (cold water only) to the kitchen—the only water to be used for drinking and cooking. Solder contains lead, and when two sections are "sweated" together, some of the solder seeps into the interior portion of the pipe. The water leaches out small amounts of lead, which, if drunk, will eventually end up in the body tissues of the user. This is perhaps not enough to produce overt lead poisoning, but when it is consumed every day, year after year, the possibility exists that even sublethal doses could have a marked (even though subtle) effect. Researchers are just now discovering how extensive the adverse effects of lead poisoning from automobile fumes are, and perhaps those same effects may arise from drinking solder-contaminated water. The use of flare fittings rather than soldered joints costs a little more, but because only a few were used, the small additional expense was well worth it. Such precautions, of course, need to be taken only with the *drinking* water; other uses

—washing, laundry, toilet, and so on—could certainly employ sweated-joint copper or plastic plumbing.

Another system that I spent a good deal of time thinking about is the electrical wiring. As of now, there is no evidence that electromagnetic radiation from household wiring is physiologically harmful, although some researchers are raising questions (as discussed in Chapter 5). But because the possibility exists that detrimental effects will be discovered, and because I intrinsically am wary of living in an environment inundated by what essentially is unnatural radiation, I chose to eliminate as much of it as possible.

Two basic kinds of wiring are used in homes today. One is a metal-enclosed cable called "BX." The other is plastic-clad cable, the most common form of wiring in houses built since 1960. I chose the metal-covered BX because it is more likely to shield the home from wire-induced electromagnetic radiation.

One last household "system" that required research was the insulation. In these days of increasing fuel costs, extensive insulation is a necessity. But which of the scores of brands should be installed, and should it be fiberglass, loose-fill, rigid-foam, foamed-in-place, or what?

To clarify a most complicated subject, I compiled the following list:

INSULATION

POROUS, BLOWN-IN, OR POURED-IN:
1. Blown-in fiberglass and rock wool
2. Blown-in cellulosic
3. Poured-in vermiculite and perlite

FOAMED-IN-PLACE:
4. Urea-formaldehyde

RIGID
5. Polystyrene (Styrofoam) and polyurethane

BATTS AND BLANKETS:
6. Fiberglass and rock wool

---

1. *Blown-in fiberglass and rock wool:* This is usually blown into walls of preexisting structures, and it is installed only by professionals. Dust from the material may well be dispersed throughout the house during installation, so windows should be open and the family should spend a day or two elsewhere. Once the blow-in process is completed, the particles likely will settle quickly or blow out open windows, although I know of no studies that have verified this. Because blown-in material is generally used in homes already built, it was inappropriate for mine.

2. *Blown-in cellulosic:* This is made from salvaged, ground-up newspapers to which boric acid, borax, and ammonium sulfate have been added as fire retardants. I would not permit cellulosic insulation in my home. For one thing, the retardant chemicals may be corrosive to metals with which they come in contact—pipes, ducts, electric wires. A more immediate source of concern to the chemically sensitive person is that the newspaper material is dustlike, and it can easily waft through crevices to cause allergic reactions. And if that weren't enough, the residual newsprint and the old ink now has the opportunity to aerosolize. Further, according to the Department of Housing and Urban Development, the fire-resistant-treatment materials ordinarily in cellulosic fiber may break down in hot attics and contaminate the whole household.[6] One physician recently reported that he was called for a consultation regarding a house in which members of a family developed sudden allergy symptoms of such severity they couldn't stand to stay in the house. He checked all the usual problem areas, he reported, "but there was something else causing trouble. It finally appeared to be the insulation that had been poured in the attic—a recycled wastepaper fiber with a fire retardant added to it. . . . It will have to be removed, and it will be a lot harder to take out of the attic than it was to put in."

One of my own patients developed a chronic cough the day cellulosic fiber was installed. Another eventually had to sell her home because of the constant headaches and rhinitis that developed from cellulose sensitivity.

On top of all these hazards, according to *Consumer Reports,* despite the fire-retardant chemicals, the material will burn anyway. In an article titled "Cellulose Insulation: Proceed with Caution," the magazine had this to say:

> Cellulose is not the only type of insulation that will burn, but cellulose made from reprocessed paper presents the greatest safety hazard in our view. . . . The increase in cellulose production brought on a major problem in quality control, both in manufacturing and installing. Existing safety standards are difficult to enforce. . . . For now we think *you should make cellulose installation your last choice.*[7]

3. *Vermiculite and perlite:* These materials, in their natural state, contain water in their molecular structure. When the materials are heated, the water expands, forming "expanded vermiculite" and "expanded perlite." From a petrochemical viewpoint, neither is polluting, but because of the lack of size uniformity, much of the material is microscopic, and can easily float through the air to be carried down into the small crevices of the lungs. Silicosis, a disease caused by breathing siliceous material, is a possibility. Therefore, neither vermiculite nor perlite should be used except in masonry cavities that are permanently sealed with cement.

4. *Foamed-in-place urea-formaldehyde:* This is used both in existing structures and in those under construction, and it is installed only by professionals. It seemed at first to look good, especially when I found that the propellant used to convert the liquid to a foam is nitrogen, an inert and harmless gas. But then I learned that when the insulation is heated to about 97 degrees F.—which is likely in attics and within dark-colored outside walls in summertime—the foam releases small amounts of formaldehyde, linked to an increasing number of headache, allergy, and respiratory problems. In a 1978 article, the *Medical Tribune* reported that Russian studies have shown that factory workers exposed daily to formalde-

hyde at a concentration of 1.6 ppm (parts per million) became irritable and insomniac. Yet one family in Connecticut was found to be living in a home atmosphere of 27 ppm. "Another victim was still breathing a concentration of 15 ppm three months after installation but was not able to smell it, even though the odor threshold is reportedly well under 1 ppm," said the *Tribune*. One Binghamton, New York, psychiatrist, Dr. Albert Wolkoff, was unable to work in his office for several weeks after urea-formaldehyde was foamed into his walls. Whenever he tried, his eyes, throat, and nose became irritated and his head began to ache. In 1978 Nancy Pappas, a writer for the Hartford *Courant,* uncovered more than twenty families suffering from formaldehyde-induced illness in Connecticut alone.[8]

In December of 1979, Massachusetts became the first state to ban urea-formaldehyde foam for insulation.

Occupants of mobile homes, for some reason (perhaps because of the structures' tightness or metal construction), seem to be particularly vulnerable to formaldehyde outgassing.[9] In 1978 Peter A. Breysse, a University of Washington assistant professor in environmental health who had been studying the problem, reported that many mobile-home owners had been undergoing treatment for "mysterious ailments" for years with little success, since neither patient nor doctor was aware of formaldehyde exposure. He pointed out that "infants, who are housebound, and elderly people, often suffering from heart or lung ailments, are especially vulnerable."[10] Needless to say, I bypassed formaldehyde insulation.

5. *Rigid polystyrene (Styrofoam) and polyurethane:* These should be used only outside of the house as a masonry insulator. When burned, both materials release extremely toxic fumes, and polyurethane, when heated only a little above the boiling point, releases flammable gas.

6. *Batts and blankets:* These are flexible, fibrous sheets of fiberglass, usually attached to aluminum foil or to paper. Batts come in precut rectangles, blankets in long rolls, both in widths to fit between studs.

I quickly eliminated kraft-paper-backed batts and rolls for my home. The paper is adhered to the fiberglass with asphalt, and the idea of being surrounded for years by slowly evaporating petrochemicals makes me very uneasy.

And finally I decided against aluminum-backed fiberglass. Had my site been within a city or close to such electromagnetic sources as television stations or microwave-relay towers, I would have seriously considered the metal-backed insulation to act as sort of a cocoon, as a Faraday cage, insulating my family, to some extent, from the radiation. But because I'm in an area relatively free from electronic smog, I feel that it's better *not* to be surrounded by such a buffer. And perhaps there are unknown benefits to be derived from exposure to natural radiation, to the rhythms of the universe (as discussed in Chapter 5). In addition, I don't want to be more or less trapped inside my home with the radiation being generated by the house current and the various devices it runs.

That leaves unbacked fiberglass. Backing, however, performs an essential function. It acts as a vapor barrier, restricting the movement of water vapor. If moisture-laden air from a heated room is able to work its way into the insulation, as it moves closer to the winter-cold outer wall it condenses, eventually to rot the framework and sheathing, and to provide an ideal place for massive amounts of mold.

So the material I finally decided on is plain fiberglass, friction fit with no attached vapor barrier; a vapor barrier of polyethylene is *separately* applied to the room side of the studs. For ceiling and floor insulation, I used specially designed Trus-joints. (For those who plan to build their own home, engineering drawings are included in Appendix B.)

Foundation

With the systems and insulation questions settled, I moved on, still working closely with the architect and engineer, to the foundation.

From a health standpoint, the foundation design presents two areas of concern: water (keeping it outside) and termites (guarding against them without resorting to poisons).

My house was designed to have no basement. Nevertheless, because I built into the side of a hill, and because I have a five-foot crawl space, I was faced with some of the same problems as those who build full basements. One of the most important steps before excavating for a new home is to find out what's down there, under the surface. You do that by taking test borings, or simply by digging a series of holes. You might find a rock ledge, for example, and you'll know that if you put the house there, the cost will go up because of the expense of removing the rock. With test borings you also will know how high the water table is; if you have a spring seeping a few feet under the surface, that should give you even more pause before you add a basement. Keeping a basement or deep crawl space dry is enough of a headache without adding the problems connected with high water tables.

Most houses need to be protected by drain tile, and the most common now used is four-inch PVC pipe with holes into which water can drain, then run off, away from the foundation to a sewer, a lower part of the property, or a dry well. In my case, natural drainage might lead one to assume that the slope would handle any subsurface water that might impinge on the foundation. Nevertheless, to be doubly certain, I insisted on having drain tile installed. The use of perforated pipe, in what is called *perifoundation* drainage, allows any water that has seeped below the ground level to flow smoothly and without obstruction around the building and away (see Appendix B). Without such precautions, water may dam up behind the foundation wall and create a powerful hydrostatic pressure, ultimately working its way between the blocks (in cement-block construction) or under the wall at the point where it rests on its base, then into the basement or crawl space. Incidentally, when the pipe is laid, I suggest that the homeowner be out there in the yard, watching. (You may not understand what you're looking at, but that fact should remain hidden.) Because everything is buried, workers sometimes tend to become sloppy, misaligning the pipe or paying too little attention to the grade of the slope. An accurate slope to the pipe is critical if water is to drain properly.

The underground section of the foundation wall itself must be dampproofed. All foundations, whether poured concrete or block, contain porous material that to some extent allows the passage of water through the wall into the house interior. What is required is a dense *cementous* material, cement so finely milled that it is water-impervious. One excellent nontoxic product (the only brand I know) is Thoroseal. It is 100 percent cementous, contains no petrochemicals, and will last the life of the building, which is not the case with primitive, tar-type waterproofing. (In fact, it is so nontoxic that a friend used it to line concreted tanks in which he raised trout. Trout are extremely sensitive to the smallest quantities of pollution. His thrived.)

The use of this cementous material will also make the foundation termite-resistant by plugging any cracks and defects that might be present. One very important point: The joint between the foundation and footing (see Appendix B) must be "coved" with a paste of Thoroseal. This is the joint that would be the first to give trouble.

A further comment concerning potential foundation cracks: A poured concrete foundation is the best since it is reinforced with steel, and except for the joints at the ends of the sections, it is a monolithic structure. Each section is poured independently. (It is a poor construction practice to pour the entire foundation at once because slight shrinkage of the concrete when it hardens would produce cracks.) Cracks between sections are "controlled," in the sense that when one section hardens, another is poured up against it.

The problem now arises as to how the entrance of moisture and termites through the seam can be prevented. If the seam is covered with Thoroseal or any other substance, the natural expansion of the foundation with temperature change will simply reestablish the seam, and the material will crack. Thomas Ryan, a Troy, New York, structural engineer (of Ryan-Biggs Engineering), and I worked out an expandable construction joint of copper.

In regard to block construction, despite the fact that the blocks have been cast at the factory, shrinkage will still occur. And because a block foundation is not as strong as poured concrete, cracking of the foundation is more common. Ryan and I worked out a modified block foundation that encompasses some elements of the poured concrete and is a general improvement on the standard block construction.

For foundation color one can use a coat of pretinted masonry cement mixed with portland cement in a ratio of three shovelfuls of portland to one 50- to-70-pound bag of tinted masonry cement. Precolored Thoroseal can also be used here, but the selection of colors is limited. Masonry supply houses—especially cement-block manufacturers—can supply the pigment by itself, and the mason can mix to the desired color.

I recommend this whole complicated procedure to all mold-wary home builders. Skimp elsewhere in the construction if you want, but take every precaution you can against basement or crawl-space dampness.

One other aspect of foundations that demands additional thought is termite control. Not long ago termites in the United States were limited to the warm sections. Today they can be found almost anywhere in the country except the Canadian border and Alaska.[11]

The key phrase for termite control in building a healthy house is *prevention without poison*. The standard procedure for protection against termites is to dump vast quantities of powerful insecticides into the ground around the foundation, and even to paint supporting timbers with it. Consult nearly any book on house construction and the so-called authority will probably recommend saturating the ground with poison. It is a dangerous solution at best. Chlordane, the biocide most commonly used, breaks down so slowly that it stays in the ground for years, killing not only the termites but everything else as well, even working its way into the groundwater and fuming up through the foundation and into the house.

One needn't resort to poisons, although if all else fails, and you *must,* you could use cryolite, a fluoride compound used in the manufacturing of aluminum. Although it is very toxic, it produces virtually no fumes. Nonpoison alternatives, however, are just as effective, if carried out during construction. The common American termite cannot stand being dry and and it cannot eat through concrete (although it can squeeze through cracks $\frac{1}{32}$ inch wide). And since a termite's home is in the ground, to travel from there, over the concrete, and into the house without drying out, it must build tunnels— tan-colored and $\frac{1}{4}$ to $\frac{1}{2}$ inch around—that can be seen and destroyed. Foundation walls should extend at least a foot above the earth, and crawl spaces should be at least four feet high so that the foundation can be easily inspected.

Incidentally, the workmen should be cautioned against burying waste wood, a fairly common practice with some builders. It's easier than hauling it off to the dump, but buried construction wood is like candy to termites. And when a newly established colony has devoured that supply, what's the next nearest source?

One other termite preventive is chemically treated wood. It's used for the base of the house, mainly the sill plate (the main member that rests atop the whole surface of the foundation wall), primarily because it is not susceptible to wood rot and is termite-resistant. The two substances most often used in the United States for wood protection (from both termites and rot) are creosote and CCA (inorganic salts of copper, chromium and arsenic). Creosote should *not* be used; CCA *should* be. Creosote is an odoriferous, oily liquid obtained from wood tar. It takes years to dry out completely, and all that time it may be fuming up into the house, producing allergic symptoms in the occupants. Dr. Randolph tells of one of his patients who was forced to sell his home because of the odors of creosote-impregnated floor supports.

CCA, on the other hand, is a stable, protective salt forced deep into the wood under high pressure. The best-known brands are Koppers' Wolmanized Pressure-Treated Lumber* and Osmose. Although the chemical names sound formidable, the compound, which has been used as a telephone-pole preservative since 1938 (many forty-year-old poles are still standing) and for dock pilings, produces no pollution. And even when buried it has virtually no susceptibility to leaching because the CCA is chemically combined with the wood.[12] Americans building homes in tropical climates, in fact, are now beginning to use CCA-treated wood exclusively, inside and out, because of its resistance both to termites and to rot.

Metal termite shields, designed to prevent termites from building tunnels up foundations, are also common, particularly in the south. But they are difficult to install properly, and authorities are unenthusiastic regarding their practicability.

With the questions of the foundation and the main support settled, my architect, engineer and I moved on to other components.

Roof

With proper ventilation, the exposed surfaces of roofs present no health problems, even though they are constructed of such substances as asphalt, which is noxious to the chemically sensitive. One caution: A window overlooking a flat tarred roof will receive fumes in the summer. A slate or metal roof will solve the problem. (Plastic roofs are new and so far are unpredictable.)

Roof ventilation is important not only to sweep away irritating fumes, but to help keep the whole-house temperature down during hot summer days, so the need for artificial cooling is less. A light color is desirable for the same reason; it can reflect some 70 percent of the sun's

---

* For a brochure on Wolmanized wood, write Forest Products Division, Koppers Company, Inc., Pittsburgh, PA 15219.

heat rays. Architectural designer Ken Kern points out that the two principles of a cool roof—air flow and color —are illustrated by the Arab's tent, which "as a functional shelter-form reflects and deflects the hottest sun on earth. The Arab tent actually consists of two separate tents. The upper one is white and acts as a reflective layer; the lower one, inside it, is additionally protected by the blanket of moving air in between." He also points out that the attic exhaust fan, the modern equivalent, is an artificial cooling aid easy to install and to operate.[13] And of course the ridge vent uses natural convection without having to resort to fans.

Exterior Siding

If the outer walls are separated from the interior with vaporproof barriers, the siding material and its protective finish should have little effect on the inhabitants. In extreme cases, the sun could volatilize the finish and the fumes could drift into the home through open windows. But I know of only one such incident, and that was when creosote was used as an exterior stain—an outmoded, impractical, and noisome practice. If a vapor barrier is not present, fumes from the asphalt-impregnated building felt (which is laid beneath the sheathing as an extra barrier to moisture and air) would continually seep into the home. This would be an intolerable situation.

The only other health question is that of metal siding, and whether or not a Faraday-cage effect is acceptable. For the same reason I avoided aluminum-backed insulation, I rejected aluminum siding; I wanted natural radiation to enter and man-made waves to exit.

Windows

Sunlight streaming through conventional glass is not the same as that coming in through a window of plastic.

Window glass filters out all wavelengths of light shorter than about 3,200 angstroms—the ultraviolet rays, the rays necessary for tanning. Some plastics allow them to pass.

Does it matter? Nobody knows; almost no solid, long-term research has been done on the health effects of light on human beings (except, of course, that involved in the production of vitamin D). Much of the work that has been done was accomplished by pioneer photobiologist John Ott, director of the Light Research Institute in Sarasota, Florida, and he believes that anyone who uses conventional window glass in his home is depriving himself of the full, healthful effects of the sun.[14] With virtually no hard scientific evidence to go on, I nevertheless tend to suspect that Ott is right. But that suspicion wasn't strong enough to cause me to use plastic instead of glass in my home.

I did, however, use it in an enclosed porch. The plastic was set in removable aluminum frames so that in the summer the area could be screened, and in winter enclosed by plastic, allowing the porch to be flooded with sunlight rich in ultraviolet all year round. Now I have the luxury of tanning in the middle of the winter.

Caulking

In a house that is adequately insulated, the major heat loss occurs in the cracks around windows and doors; therefore, thorough caulking is essential, both to save money and to help keep the inside humidity level high during the dry days of winter. Two suggestions here: that you use "double-component polyurethane" (for durability) and that you employ a caulking specialist rather than leave the job to the general contractor; the cost will be the same, and the work will be superior. (If you decide not to employ a specialist, an easy-to-apply "one-component polyurethane" is available; the common, off-the-shelf varieties are not recommended because they release vapors for months, and perhaps longer.)

Studs

About three years ago the Department of Housing and Urban Development and the U.S. Forest Service developed Com-Ply two-by-four studs. The process consists of grinding up whole logs (bark, core, branches and all), bonding the mixture with a phenolic resin under heat and pressure, then gluing on veneer facings.[15] When *Popular Science* featured the new material, this is what one reader reported to the editor:

> I feel I should share an experience I've had with one resin-bonded wood product.
>
> After incorporating larger-than-usual quantities of composition board in a recent major basement remodeling, I discovered that about five to twenty percent of the visitors to the completed recreation room develop allergic reactions, ranging from mild to severe eye tearing or burning. Only a complete periodic ventilation alleviated the problem. Covering or otherwise sealing some of the particle board helped as well.
>
> Since these reactions were apparently caused by resin vapors from the particle board, I wonder aloud if the same resin or allergy-causing resin agent is used in Com-Ply products. I would strongly recommend that potential Com-Ply customers investigate this matter before constructing an entire house to which they may be allergic.[16]

My recommendation is even stronger: Don't even consider it.

The standard interior wall, gypsum board (also known as plasterboard, wallboard, dry wall, or Sheetrock), has also reportedly irritated some ultrasensitive patients, but whether the trouble arises from the plaster, the glue that binds the surface paper, or the joint compound (that hides board junctions) I haven't been able to determine. There have been reports of formaldehyde outgassing from wallboards used in apartment constructions[17] and problems caused by wallboard fumes among El Paso, Texas, schoolchildren,[18] but I've been unable to verify them.

However, joint compounds (and spackling compounds) have as their ingredients a number of toxic substances, according to a team from the Environmental Science Laboratory of Mount Sinai School of Medicine in New York City. Among them: talc, quartz, feldspar, mica, clay, calcite, dolomite, and plaster of paris—all, say team members, implicated in respiratory diseases. In addition, nine of the ten products tested by the researchers contained asbestos fibers. Said team member A. N. Rohl, as the report was published:

> Even the incidental exposure—for example, of a day or so —to levels *less* than occupational exposures have been shown to produce fatal tumors. Our problem is that we haven't come to grips with the lower end of the dose-response curve. We just don't know exactly how low an exposure level can induce tumor formation, so we have to look at exposure very conservatively.[19]

Rohl suggested that do-it-yourselfers take three main precautions when installing gypsum board:

1. Avoid raising dust while working with spackling, patching, and jointing compounds. If possible, buy premixed products.
2. Smooth over moist compounds with a wet cloth instead of sanding them smooth after they harden.
3. Approved respirators should be worn to filter out whatever dust is raised.

Interior Walls

For most of the interior walls in my house, I used wood panels and tongue-and-groove planking, some in its natural state, some with a coating of polyurethane. The main reason is that wood is *hygroscopic,* absorbing moisture from the room atmosphere. This imparts a fairly decent antistatic effect to its surface, discouraging the accumulation of charges and allowing negative ions to remain in the air.

Because softwoods (pine, spruce, and especially cedar and redwood) contain resins that are volatile and remain so for years after installation—resins that have the same biochemical effect on sensitized individuals as petroleum-product vapors—I installed only hardwoods, birch, beech, and teak, on both the walls and trim. In the closets I placed plywood. So far as I can tell, plywood causes no major problems. The fresh, lumberyard aroma soon gasses out, and the binding cement appears not to be troublesome. Plywood-panel wall glue or contact cement, however, should be avoided; blind nailing is mandatory.

I also avoided:

Cork: Since particles are bound with noxious petrochemicals, cork walls can be a major polluter.

Vinyl tile and sheets: (1) Plastic holds an electrical charge; (2) sunlight falling on the surface may cause depolymerization; and (3) it requires gluing that may itself add to the household pollution.

Imitation wood (such as melamine plastic with printed wood grain): It, too, holds electrical charges.

Wallpaper: (1) It may flake, causing cellulose particles to add to the air pollution; (2) the paste is suspect— it may include unlabeled anti-insect and antifungal chemicals; and (3) the plastic coating of some types could hold charges and contribute to the destruction of the electrical environment.

Pressed wood (particle board, chipboard): These products are made from varying sizes of wood chips mixed with urea-formaldehyde resins and bonded under pressure. The resins, tending to volatilize formaldehyde, have caused major problems[20] (as discussed in the section on insulation).

In certain sections of the house, I used brick and tile on the walls—both superior materials. Stucco and stone would have been equally acceptable. I also selected flat, simple baseboards with no crevices to hold dust.

Floors

For the subflooring, I chose plywood exclusively, even though it is somewhat more expensive than commonly employed particle board; I wanted no formaldehyde fumes seeping up from between the floorboards. Subflooring must be both nailed and *glued* to the floor joists to get a cohesive "monolithic" floor of maximum strength and durability.

Some builders treat the roof similarly, as did mine. I selected Gulf's Flooring and General Construction Adhesive, which comes in an applicator cartridge. I preliminarily tried out the glue, and after it dried fully I could detect no odor, nor could my sensitive patients. I still prefer blind nailing for the *interior* panels, just to be safe, but because the subflooring and roof are actually on the *exterior* surfaces of the house (bathed in air currents of the crawl space and vented attic), I feel that the risk is minimal.

The floors themselves are either hardwood (no resinous vapors) or ceramic tile. I planned to surface the hardwood with three coats of polyurethane, which gasses out quickly, leaving a hard finish that never needs to be waxed, but I found that most prestained hardwood floorings come coated with wax, which makes application of polyurethane impossible. So one must either use unfinished flooring and then apply the stain, or find a supplier of flooring that is already coated with polyurethane.

For the tile sections of the house, I originally planned to lay terrazzo, but I learned that it is porous, and that to guard against staining, it would have to be sealed, and usually waxed—which, of course, is unacceptable. So I switched to a tile with a glazed surface—impervious and permanent. I chose Structural Stoneware so I wouldn't have to sacrifice aesthetics for function. (Nonglazed, dense "quarry tile" is also impervious to stain, requiring neither wax nor sealer.) For those who insist on vinyl tiles or vinyl sheet goods, a waterbase cement is recommended.

The only floor coverings in the whole house are small washable cotton throwrugs in the bedrooms and bath, and oriental rugs, which are easily removed for cleaning. No wall-to-wall carpets, no linoleum, no plastic, cork or rubber, for the reasons given in Chapter 6. I wanted to cut down as much as possible on dust, vapors, and ion attraction. (By the way, radiant-heated floors surfaced with floor coverings are particularly bad; the heat will slowly volatilize materials in the cement and covering, producing fumes possibly for years.)

Fireplace

This stumped me for quite awhile. I knew that burning fireplaces can puff at times, discharging quantities of smoke and gas into the living room. I knew that an unlit fireplace, if the wind is right, can coat the room with soot. I knew that smoke from a furnace chimney can be blown down an adjacent fireplace chimney into the living quarters. I knew that a fireplace is an atavistic anachronism that gives a lot of charm and little heat, that in most cases it pulls more heat from the house and blows it up the chimney than it adds, that the air drawn into a fireplace to fuel the flame causes a vacuum that pulls cold air into the house through window and door cracks, effectively cooling the whole house except for the spot directly before the flame. I knew that shortly after you light up most fireplaces the furnace turns on. And if all this weren't sufficient reason to exclude fireplaces from any sensible house design, I knew that they lower the relative humidity (from the outside air being sucked in), drying respiratory tracts of anyone foolish enough to have one, and that fireplaces distort the electrical environment as well.

Nevertheless, I wanted one.

What I needed was a fireplace that heats the air inside the room, yet uses outside air for burning. After some search, I discovered a number of such systems. The front of these fireplaces are covered by close-fitting glass doors, effectively sealing off air from the room. The air for the fire comes from an outside vent, usually directly behind the logs. Above the fire three concentric tubes act as a heat exchanger to trap the heat that is headed up the chimney. So what the fireplace employs is a totally independent circulation; no smoke ever enters the room, and no warm and humidified air from the room ever goes up the chimney.

So now I can sit in my twentieth-century living room before my caveman campfire, and I'm content.

Kitchen

The most important item here is a hood and exhaust fan above the range (electric, of course, not gas), large enough to quickly remove vaporized oils and smoke before they can permeate the house. Cabinets are of hardwood and plywood, prefinished at the factory and allowed to age and gas out before installation. Again, no particle board was used because of the outgassing of formaldehyde. (Metal cabinets would also have been acceptable.) The countertops are of ceramic—easy to clean and nonabsorbent. Stainless steel would also have been a good choice, but plastic laminates, such as Formica, would not, since they customarily are cemented to particle board. One substitute I've used is plywood with a "stain grade" wood veneer, surfaced with three coats of polyurethane. It's almost as hard as plastic laminate, and I much prefer its appearance.

"Chopping-block" counter surfaces are poor; they are always wet, and as they age, the cracks between the wood strips open to allow mold to flourish.

Bath

Here, I used hard glass tile (durable and nonporous), closely fit with a narrow grouted portion for easy cleaning. Ions produced by the rushing shower, together with the ceramic tiles, produce a good electrostatic environment.

Sauna

I rejected an electric sauna, of course, because of the enormous quantity of both electromagnetic waves and positive ions given off.[21] Instead, I selected an imported Scandinavian wood-burning unit designed so that the wood is fed into the fire from a different room, eliminating the possibility of air pollution. The interior is lined with aspen, a wood that is nonresinous.

Yard

Most home designers give far too little thought to landscaping. And when the occupant finally does get around to noticing that his new castle looks as if it's built on an Appalachian strip mine, his decisions on what to put where are based solely on aesthetics, not on function. A tree would look nice here. A couple of bushes there. Another tree there, and some flowers someplace—there? Both beauty and function are important, and the most important function from a health point of view is shade control, to eliminate the need for artificial summer cooling as much as possible.

A few deciduous trees provide generous shade for the house in the dog days of summer; yet, remarkably, at just the right time, they lose their leaves so sunlight can stream through their bare branches to warm the home as the frigid days of late fall move in. Strategically located trees, say landscape engineers, can actually reduce heating and cooling costs by a third or more.

The aesthetics of planting are a matter between the owner and his nurseryman. But here are a few functional points a home designer might bear in mind:

- When planning tree sites, think of what the trees

will be when matured—how large, how high up to the
first branches, what the roots might do to foundations,
what other vegetation will be shaded.

• A mature tree close to the house shades it from mid-
morning to midafternoon. One farther away might block
the light of dawn, the sky of sunset. Is that desirable?

• Evergreens set too near the house will block warming winter sun, but a row of them set across the yard to
the north can act as an effective windbreak, reducing
heat loss and discouraging drifting snow. Hedges can
also act as snow fences.

• Shrubs usually are planted too close to the house.
They impede air, which in turn slows evaporation, often
causing mold conditions along the lower portions of the
house. Bare-trunked trees and grass allow the breeze to
flow.

• Thick plantings of hedges, bushes, and trees on the
side toward the road can help block traffic sounds, another form of pollution. The viscous leaves also act as a
general filter, trapping some of the dust stirred up by
passing vehicles.

The design of a healthy house is, as you have seen, a
series of compromises. The home I have built is, within
the limits of practicality and aesthetics, the closest possible to a truly healthy house. Nevertheless, it's not per-
fect. An east wind still occasionally carries with it
Hudson River Valley smog. The dog continues to scatter
his dander around the living room. The food-processor
motor adds its touch of vaporized lubricating oil. The oriental rug—a significant compromise that I pondered for
quite a time—wafts up its dust every time I cross it. I
throw open the windows to clear out the dust with a
sweet, clean breeze of fall, and fill my home with ragweed pollen.

You, too, when you design your house, will compromise. And building a house that won't be detrimental to
your health—locating it in an area with an atmosphere
as free from chemical and electrical pollutants as possible, furnishing that home with materials innocuous to

sensitivities, stocking it with as few man-made chemicals as possible—is, at the least, an inconvenience. But for the highly sensitive individual, the principles given in these chapters should be followed as closely as possible. For the person who has no obvious sensitivities at all, though, some of the suggestions can be relaxed. But beware. As the introduction emphasizes, *everyone* is environmentally susceptible.

Appendix A
Checklist to Identify Health Hazards

When someone moves into a house and immediately becomes ill, he usually knows that something is wrong with his surroundings, even though he may not know exactly what. But usually the maladies that an unhealthy house bestow develop slowly. And they're so removed from any obvious toxins in the environment that it often takes an extraordinarily aware person to connect strange and varied symptoms with cause.

The following pages are designed to help you find out if you have developed sensitivities to your environment. The first section is a checklist of symptoms that an unhealthy house can bring about. This is followed by a questionnaire that, with the aid of your physician, will help define your problem—the first major step to finding a solution.

And even if you can't entirely eliminate your problems, it's important to know *why* you're ill. If you know what is wrong and try to avoid the source of the problem, even if you're only partially successful, you'll feel enormously better. As Theron Randolph puts it, "Acute reactions of *known* causation are infinitely more endurable than chronic illness of *unknown* origin."[1]

Start with the following section. Think back over the last few weeks to see if you've experienced any of the difficulties in the left-hand list, then check one of the right-hand columns. If you think you *may* have the problem but aren't sure, check the "?" column.

Symptoms of an Unhealthy Environment

Test yourself for symptoms that may indicate health hazards within the home. If you think you may have a problem but are uncertain, check the "?" column.

NERVE AND MUSCLE PROBLEMS

	YES	?	NO
1. Fainting	—	—	—
2. Blurred vision	—	—	—
3. Unexplained hyperactivity	—	—	—
4. Headache	—	—	—
5. Dizziness	—	—	—

MOOD CHANGES

	YES	?	NO
1. Unexplained anxiety	—	—	—
2. Unwarranted excitability	—	—	—
3. Unexplained irritability	—	—	—
4. Hostility	—	—	—
5. Aggression	—	—	—
6. Insomnia	—	—	—
7. Restlessness	—	—	—
8. Difficulty concentrating	—	—	—
9. Difficulty thinking	—	—	—
10. Mental confusion	—	—	—
11. Grogginess	—	—	—
12. Decreased reading comprehension	—	—	—
13. Forgetfulness	—	—	—
14. Difficulty recalling words	—	—	—
15. Depression	—	—	—
16. Loss of interest in work or former activities or hobbies	—	—	—
17. Crying spells	—	—	—
18. Tendency for fixed ideas; recycling or repeating of ideas	—	—	—
19. Antisocial behavior	—	—	—
20. Thoughts of suicide	—	—	—

ORGANS AND SYSTEMS PROBLEMS   YES   ?   NO

1. Skin
   Rashes   ___ ___ ___
   Excessive perspiration   ___ ___ ___
2. Eyes
   Burning   ___ ___ ___
   Itching   ___ ___ ___
   Excessive tearing   ___ ___ ___
   Feeling of heaviness and pressure within eyes   ___ ___ ___
3. Ears
   Dizziness (Menière's syndrome)   ___ ___ ___
   Decreased hearing   ___ ___ ___
   Buzzing in ears (tinnitus)   ___ ___ ___
   "Plugged" ears (swollen eustachian tubes)   ___ ___ ___
4. Nose
   Nasal obstruction   ___ ___ ___
   Sinus congestion   ___ ___ ___
   Sneezing (Rubbing nose upward is a sign of
      allergy)   ___ ___ ___
5. Throat
   Hoarseness   ___ ___ ___
   "Itching" throat (leading to clucking sounds)   ___ ___ ___
   Sore throat   ___ ___ ___
   Excessive mucus   ___ ___ ___
6. Lungs
   Wheezing   ___ ___ ___
   Coughing   ___ ___ ___
7. Cardiovascular
   Palpitations   ___ ___ ___
   Flushing   ___ ___ ___
8. Gastrointestinal
   Nausea   ___ ___ ___
   Loss of appetite   ___ ___ ___
   Voracious appetite or sudden weight gain
   (5 pounds in 2 days)   ___ ___ ___
   Chronic obesity   ___ ___ ___
   Excessive thirst   ___ ___ ___

	YES	?	NO
9. Genitourinary			
Urgent urination	___	___	___
Frequent urination	___	___	___
Bedwetting	___	___	___
Vaginal itching	___	___	___
Excessively painful menstruation	___	___	___
10. Muscular-skeletal			
Muscle soreness	___	___	___
Joint pains	___	___	___
Uncertain gait	___	___	___

GENERAL PHYSICAL PROBLEMS

	YES	?	NO
1. Fatigue (physical or mental)	___	___	___
2. Loss of former energy ("getting old")	___	___	___
3. Weakness	___	___	___
4. Edema (swelling)	___	___	___
5. Pallor	___	___	___
6. Inappropriate chilliness or excessive warmth	___	___	___
7. Excessive perspiration without fever	___	___	___
8. Unexplained fevers	___	___	___

The symptoms you just checked may fall into a pattern that up to now you haven't discerned. The quiz that follows consists of questions designed to clarify that pattern and to help uncover the cause of the symptoms.

One important step in determining the cause is to establish whether the symptoms fall into a *varying* or *constant* pattern. Varying patterns are indicated in terms of time, place, and activities:

TIME: Time of day, day of the week, seasons.

PLACE: Exclusively in the home or work environment or only in certain geographical areas.

ACTIVITIES: Only at work, or while engaged in a hobby, or when exposed to certain chemicals, or mostly after meals.

If a varying patterns exists, the likelihood is that the problem may be found in your surroundings. If a *constant* pattern exists, the cause may be more difficult to determine: You may be exposed to the source of your problem so often that the intolerable entity never is completely removed from your system, or the trouble may come from internal sources—bacteria, fungi, or other pathogenic organisms—or it may come from organic causes that have little to do with your environment. The secret is *awareness*. First, discover whether or not there *is* a problem. (Many people have lived with their low-level illness for so long they no longer know what it is to feel well or to function at full potential.) Then, after heightening that awareness, focus on the offending substances.

Narrowing the Environmental Source of Your Problem

Are you constitutionally (genetically) predisposed to develop sensitivities? "Yes" answers to even a few questions mean that you probably are. (Again, if the answer is unknown, or if you are undecided, check the middle—"?"—column.)

DURING CHILDHOOD:

	YES	?	NO
1. Did you have eczema or other skin problems (before puberty)?	——	——	——
2. Did you have colic?	——	——	——
3. Were you a feeding problem?	——	——	——
4. Were you disposed to ear infections?	——	——	——
5. Do you have a history of asthma or croup?	——	——	——
6. Do you have a history of hay fever?	——	——	——

FAMILY HISTORY:

Did your mother, father, brother, sister
or grandparents have—

1. Eczema? Who?_____	——	——	——
2. Hay fever? Who?_____	——	——	——
3. Asthma? Who?_____	——	——	——
4. Problems with foods? Who?_____	——	——	——

VARIATION BY TIME: SEASONAL INCIDENCE   YES ? NO

(Dates apply only to temperate climates; others may differ.)

Do you have symptoms or do you get worse—

1. In the spring—March to May? (Allergen could be tree pollens.)   ___ ___ ___

2. In the early summer—May to August? (Perhaps grass pollen.)   ___ ___ ___

3. In the autumn—mid-August to mid- or end of September? (May be ragweed.)   ___ ___ ___

4. From spring to first frost, with a peak from late July to frost? (Probably mold.)   ___ ___ ___

5. In the winter—mid-September to spring? (May be housedust.)   ___ ___ ___

SHORT-TIME VARIATION:

Do your symptoms occur or get worse—

Once a day?   ___ ___ ___

Regularly at a particular time of day or night?   ___ ___ ___

An hour or two after certain meals?   ___ ___ ___

The allergen could be a food. Stomach cramps at ten in the morning, for example, could indicate a response to some ingredient in the food eaten for breakfast. A postdinner depression could mean a reaction to vapors from range gas. Or a headache after gardening might mean a sensitivity to previously sprayed insecticides.

The problem might be:

MOLD

        YES ? NO

Do your symptoms occur or get worse—

1. When you are exposed to hay (fields, haystacks, barns)?   ___ ___ ___

2. When you rake dry leaves?   ___ ___ ___

3. When you are near a lawn that's being mowed?   ___ ___ ___

4. When you are in a damp basement?   ___ ___ ___

5. When you are exposed to a succession of days of damp weather?   ___ ___ ___

6. When you eat foods made by fermentation: beer, wine, sharp cheeses, sauerkraut, pickles, vinegar, mushrooms?   ___ ___ ___

7. Do you feel better when snow is on the ground? (Snow covers outside sources of mold: decayed vegetation, dry leaves, dry grass, and so on.)   ___ ___ ___

8. Are you allergic to penicillin? (Penicillin is made from mold.)   ___ ___ ___

Perhaps your problem is:

HOUSEDUST

Do your symptoms occur or get worse—

1. When the heating season starts (mid-September in the temperate zone) and get better in the spring?   ___ ___ ___

2. When the house is being swept?   ___ ___ ___

3. When the bed is being made?   ___ ___ ___

4. When you sit in overstuffed furniture?   ___ ___ ___

5. When you are in a library?   ___ ___ ___

6. When you are in the bedroom?   ___ ___ ___

7. When you arise in the morning, but then improve through the day?   ___ ___ ___

ANIMAL DANDER

Do your symptoms occur or get worse when:

1. You are exposed to mammals, such as cats, dogs, or horses?   ___ ___ ___

2. You are exposed to animal hair (rabbit, mohair, wool) in the form of blends (sweaters, gloves, liners, blankets), or rug padding, or furniture stuffing?   ___ ___ ___

3. You are exposed to feathers (in pillows or down comforters), or birds (chickens, parrots, canaries), or to someone who has been working with fowl? (Some people sensitive to fowl dander also react to eating poultry or eggs.)   ___ ___ ___

VAPORS

Do symptoms occur or get worse when you are exposed to:

1. Tobacco smoke?   ___ ___ ___

	YES	?	NO
2. Insect sprays or powders, including lawn products?	___	___	___
3. Mothproofing chemicals?	___	___	___
4. Perfumes, lotions, shampoos?	___	___	___
5. Paint fumes?	___	___	___
6. Resinous wood (Christmas trees, knotty-pine walls, cedar closets, pine-scented products, turpentine)?	___	___	___
7. Gas fumes (cooking stove, gas dryer, gas hot-water heater)?	___	___	___
8. Auto or bus fumes?	___	___	___
9. Smoke (fireplaces, furnaces, candles)?	___	___	___
10. Solvents (gasoline, kerosene, nail-polish remover, alcohol, varnish, lacquer, cleaning fluids—including visits to the cleaners)?	___	___	___
11. Polishes (furniture, floor, metal, shoe, nail)?	___	___	___
12. Lubricating greases or oils?	___	___	___
13. Room disinfectants and deodorants?	___	___	___
14. Petroleum residues (roof or road tar, or creosote from railroad ties or telephone poles), fresh newspaper ink, new leather and its polishes or dyes, weed killers?	___	___	___
15. Rubber products (gloves, mattresses, rug pads, rubber-based paints)?	___	___	___
16. Plastics (upholstery covers, bookcovers, tablecloths, window shades)?	___	___	___
17. Aerosols?	___	___	___
18. Miscellaneous: ammonia fumes (various cleaning agents), or chlorine (swimming pools, tapwater, bleaches, some scouring powders)?	___	___	___

Some people who are sensitive to certain vapors actually like to smell them, actually may get a lift from them, with a temporary relief from symptoms. Does that apply to you? Just as an alcoholic or heroin addict feels better and gets a temporary lift right after a drink or an injection, followed by an eventual letdown, vapor-sensitive people may experience *either* an immediate down or a temporary up followed by a *subsequent down* a few minutes to a few hours later. The connection might be obscure. For example, few individuals will connect such feelings as depression, tiredness, and lack of interest in the late morning with the lift that they got from breathing gasoline fumes when they stopped at the gas station on the way to work. A similar effect can occur with the ingestion of such innocuous foods as chocolate or cola drinks, or any food a person may be allergic to.

FOODS

	YES	?	NO
1. Do you frequently belch after meals?	___	___	___
2. Do you often have indigestion following meals?	___	___	___
3. Is there any food that you feel disagrees with you? What?_____	___	___	___
4. Do you often have attacks of diarrhea?	___	___	___
5. Do you suffer with cramping pains in your lower abdomen?	___	___	___
6. Have you ever been told you have mucous colitis?	___	___	___
7. Have you ever been told you have gallbladder problems?	___	___	___
8. Have you ever had acute pain in the abdomen associated with hives and itching of the skin?	___	___	___
9. Do you suspect any food of causing or aggravating your condition? What?_____	___	___	___
10. Are there any foods that you especially dislike? What?_____	___	___	___
11. Are there any foods you overindulge in or eat very frequently because you particularly *like* them? (An addiction is almost diagnostic of a food allergy.)	___	___	___
12. Is there any seasonal food (for instance, strawberries or tomatoes) in which you overindulge? What?_____	___	___	___
13. Are there any foods you find difficult to digest? What?_____	___	___	___

14. Do any foods cause nausea, vomiting, diarrhea,   YES   ?   NO
heartburn, belching, gas, cramps, hives, skin
rashes, headache?
     What?_____   ___ ___ ___

15. Do you drink or eat
___coffee more than 5 times a day?   ___ ___ ___
___ tea more than 5 times a day?   ___ ___ ___
___ cola more than 5 times a day?   ___ ___ ___
___ chocolate more than once a day?   ___ ___ ___
___ alcohol more than 3 times a day?   ___ ___ ___

COSMETICS

Do you break out in a rash when you use
cosmetics?   ___ ___ ___

     Which ones?_____

FROM THE MEDICINE CABINET

Do you react (skin rash, sneezing, and other symptoms) when you use:

1. "Deodorant" soaps?   ___ ___ ___
2. Deodorants, particularly aerosol?   ___ ___ ___
3. Feminine hygiene spray?   ___ ___ ___
4. Hair dye?   ___ ___ ___
5. Hair spray?   ___ ___ ___
6. Various skin ointments, salves, lotions, creams?   ___ ___ ___
7. Any medications?   ___ ___ ___
     What?_____

ELECTRICAL

1. Do your symptoms occur or get worse before a
rainstorm?   ___ ___ ___
2. Can you tell if it's going to rain well before it
starts because you "feel different" without any
obvious symptoms?   ___ ___ ___
3. Do you feel markedly improved at the seashore
or in the mountains?   ___ ___ ___

Now look back over the list and identify the categories that seem to be causing difficulty. With these in mind, check over the following list of common household problem entities, circling those you know or suspect may be giving you trouble.

FUELS (*petrochemicals*)
Cooking and heating gas
Kerosene
Smoke from fireplaces or furnaces
Gasoline fumes
Automobile, bus, motorboat
    exhaust
Lubricating greases and oils
Heating oil

SOLVENTS
Alcohol
Naphtha, cleaning fluids, lighter
    fluid

RUBBER
Elastic in underwear, brassieres,
    gloves
Sponge-rubber pillows,
    mattresses, rug pads
Typewriter pads
Overheated wires
Heating pads

FINISHES
Varnish, lacquer, or shellac
Floor and furniture wax
Banana oil
Rubber-based paint
Mineral-spirits-based paint
Synthetic-based paint

POLISHES
Metal
Shoe
Floor
Table

ASPHALTS AND TARS
Fumes from roof application
Asphalt roadways under summer
    sun

Dyes in cosmetics
Fumes from carbon paper,
    typewriter ribbons, fresh
    newspapers
Tar-containing ointments,
    shampoos, soaps

DEODORANTS/DISINFECTANTS
Room-deodorizing spray
Wick-type room deodorizer
Disinfectant bathroom washes
Toilet-tank deodorizers
Chlorinated water

CLEANSERS
Soap
Detergents
Ammonia
Bleaches
Scouring powder
Window cleaner

PERFUMES
Perfume or cologne
Preshave and aftershave lotions
Hair oils and tonics
Scented soaps and shampoos
Hair sprays
Incense

COSMETICS
Powder
Rouge and blushers
Lipstick
Eye shadow
Eyebrow pencil
Mascara
Eye-makeup remover
Hand and body lotion
Cold cream
Moisturizer
Nail polish

Nail-polish remover
Mineral oil
Tanning creams
Depilatories

SOFTWOOD FUMES
Pine paneling
Christmas tree
Vapors from sanding or sawing
    pine or cedar
Turpentine
Fumes from fireplace

INSECT CONTROL
Insecticides
Mothballs, flakes, crystals
Insect-repellent candles
Repellent lotions
Sprayed vegetables and fruits
Wallpaper paste
Commercially cleaned rugs
Furniture previously commercially
    stored
Secondhand mattresses and
    furniture

PLASTICS
Upholstery, tablecloths, book
    covers, handbags, pillow and
    mattress covers, curtains and
    drapes

Vapor from plastic cement
Adhesive tape
Synthetic clothing
Plastic frames for glasses
Plastic-base dentures

DRUGS
Vitamins
Tranquilizers
Analgesics
Local anesthetics
Antibiotics
Anticoagulants
Anticonvulsants
Antihistamines
Diuretics
Estrogens
Headache remedies
Laxatives
Sedatives
Steroids
Sulfonamides
Phenobarbital
Aspirin
Codeine
Demerol
Iodides
Novocaine
Penicillin
Mineral oil

(Food allergy is almost always a problem with sensitive people. But that is a different and complicated subject outside the scope of this book.)

MISCELLANEOUS
Horsehair stuffing and rug pads
Wool clothing, bedding, drapes,
    furniture

Air conditioning
Contraceptives
Douche
Marking Pens

Can you spot substances giving you trouble, and can you see a pattern emerging? Some of the symptoms—hay fever, for instance—may be treated with over-the-counter antihistamines if mild, and by a physician if severe. But by far the best treatment is avoidance. Try to change your living patterns to eliminate offending substances from your home. If a number of different entities are giving you problems, usually you needn't avoid them *all;* the elimination of one or two of the most troublesome may remove enough of the burden from your body so that your cells can handle the remaining offending substances.

If you can't seem to locate and rectify the sources of your troubles, if you're not successful in doing something about them, or if there are just too many noxious substances in your life to contend with, then it's time—equipped with your questionnaire—to visit an environmentally oriented allergist.

Appendix B
Construction Drawings

NOTE: Not everyone who reads this book is expected to build a home. However, for those who will, the following drawings are offered as an *aid to your architect, engineer, or builder*. They are technically detailed enough to quickly and graphically explain the specific suggestions of the book to the professional as well as to the interested reader.

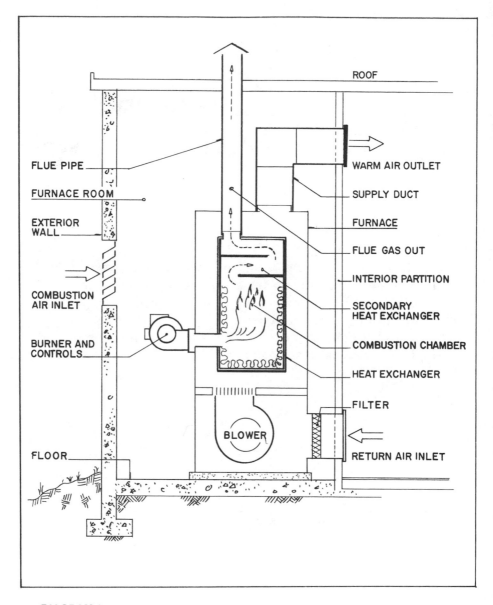

DIAGRAM 1

FORCED-AIR FURNACE, installed in a room apart from the main house. Depending on the model, the air inlet for combustion is either a screened hole in the wall (as shown) or a three-inch flexible clothes-dryer-type pipe leading to the furnace air intake.

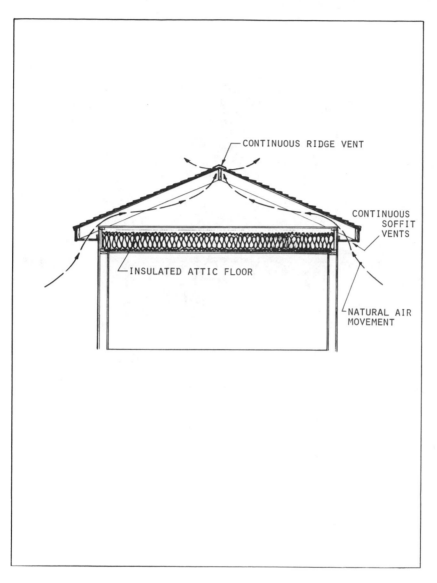

CONTINUOUS RIDGE VENT

CONTINUOUS
SOFFIT
VENTS

INSULATED ATTIC FLOOR

NATURAL AIR
MOVEMENT

DIAGRAM 2

CONTINUOUS RIDGE AND SOFFIT VENTS, allowing air to circulate through the
attic, release excessively humid or hot air (which can range upward of 175 degrees F. under the summer sun) that flows out without the aid of an exhaust fan.
Attic-floor insulation system is similar to roof (Diagram 3), except that ventilation
is not required.

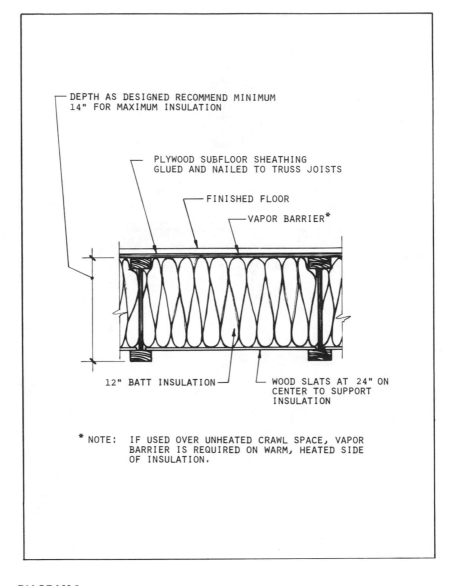

DIAGRAM 3

TRUSS JOISTS, supporting floors and roof, are designed with a lip at the bottom to hold 1×2-inch slats, which in turn support the insulation. A minimum of twelve inches of insulation is recommended for floor joists (A), fourteen inches or more

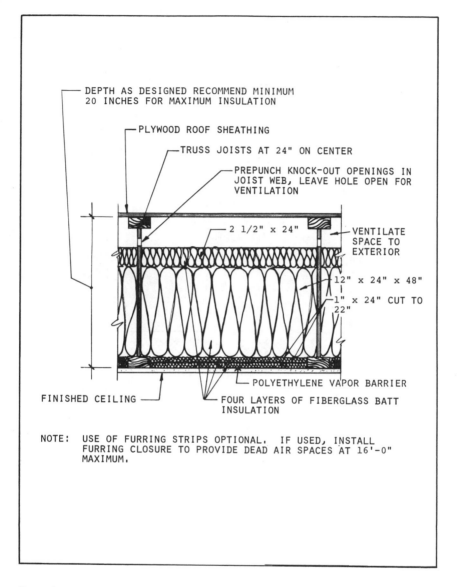

DEPTH AS DESIGNED RECOMMEND MINIMUM
20 INCHES FOR MAXIMUM INSULATION

PLYWOOD ROOF SHEATHING

TRUSS JOISTS AT 24" ON CENTER

PREPUNCH KNOCK-OUT OPENINGS IN
JOIST WEB, LEAVE HOLE OPEN FOR
VENTILATION

2 1/2" x 24"

VENTILATE
SPACE TO
EXTERIOR

12" x 24" x 48"

1" x 24" CUT TO
22"

POLYETHYLENE VAPOR BARRIER

FINISHED CEILING

FOUR LAYERS OF FIBERGLASS BATT
INSULATION

NOTE: USE OF FURRING STRIPS OPTIONAL. IF USED, INSTALL
FURRING CLOSURE TO PROVIDE DEAD AIR SPACES AT 16'-0"
MAXIMUM.

if used over unheated crawl space. Roof joists (B) differ from floor joists in two
respects: Holes allow air to ventilate along insulation to the outdoors, and insulation is thicker. Typical recommendation for maximum insulation in winter
weather similar to that of New York State: four layers of fiberglass batts, as
illustrated.

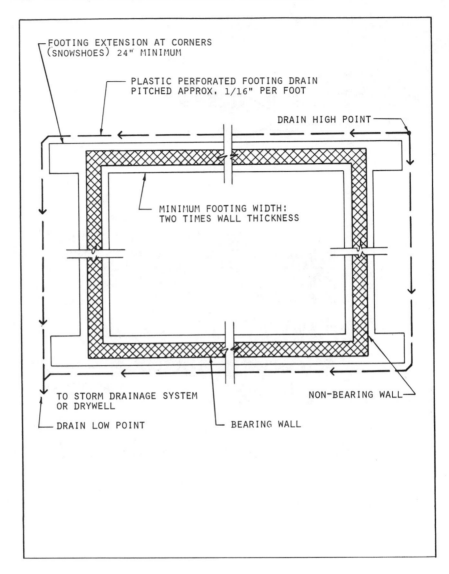

DIAGRAM 4:

PERIFOUNDATION DRAIN PATTERN, viewed from above. Water flows into the
perforated plastic footing drain at any point, then runs off to be discharged into
the drainage system at lower left. The pipe should slope at least an inch every
sixteen feet. At the foundation corners, "snowshoes" extend at least twenty-four
inches beyond the building line to strengthen corners, the weakest points in the
foundation. Conventional designs may allow underground water to undermine a
corner, and as it becomes cantilevered it can crack. The snowshoes prevent this.

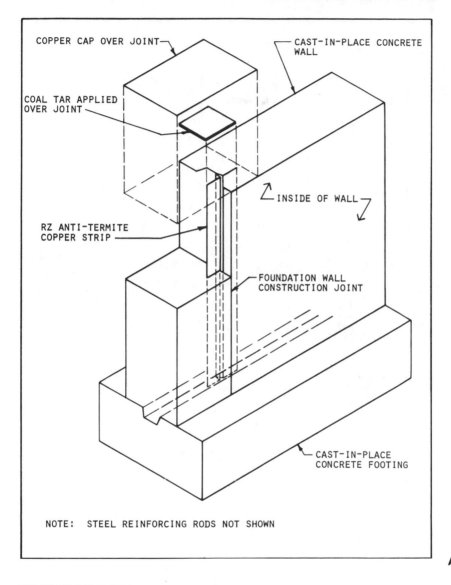

COPPER CAP OVER JOINT

CAST-IN-PLACE CONCRETE WALL

COAL TAR APPLIED OVER JOINT

INSIDE OF WALL

RZ ANTI-TERMITE COPPER STRIP

FOUNDATION WALL CONSTRUCTION JOINT

CAST-IN-PLACE CONCRETE FOOTING

NOTE: STEEL REINFORCING RODS NOT SHOWN

A

DIAGRAM 5 (A.B.C.D.):

ANTI-TERMITE JOINTS use 6½-inch-wide copper RZ strips that stretch the height of the foundation. In a poured-concrete wall (A), roofing tar seals the top, with a copper cap shielding the upper joint.

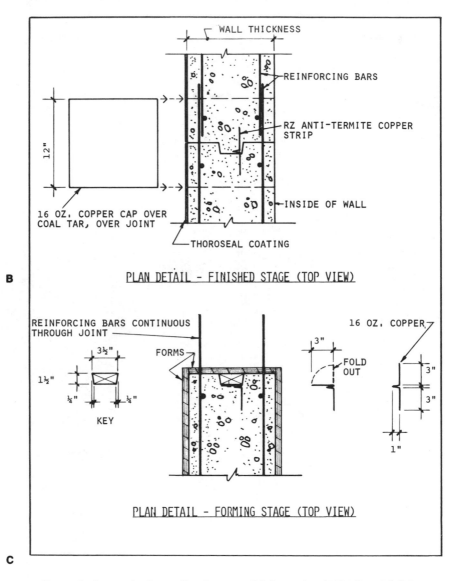

WALL THICKNESS

REINFORCING BARS

RZ ANTI-TERMITE COPPER STRIP

12"

INSIDE OF WALL

16 OZ. COPPER CAP OVER COAL TAR, OVER JOINT

THOROSEAL COATING

B

PLAN DETAIL - FINISHED STAGE (TOP VIEW)

REINFORCING BARS CONTINUOUS THROUGH JOINT

FORMS

16 OZ. COPPER

3"

FOLD OUT

3"

3½"

1½"

¼" ¼"

KEY

3"

1"

PLAN DETAIL - FORMING STAGE (TOP VIEW)

C

Concrete for a single section is poured into a standard plywood form, as shown from the top in B. The key is of 2×4-inch stock beveled for easy removal. When the concrete hardens, the copper strip is unfolded, ready to be integrated into the next section to be poured.

View C shows the RZ strip unfolded and the next section poured. Note that the horizontal reinforcing bars run through the joints. Cast-in-place sections should extend no more than forty feet without a joint.

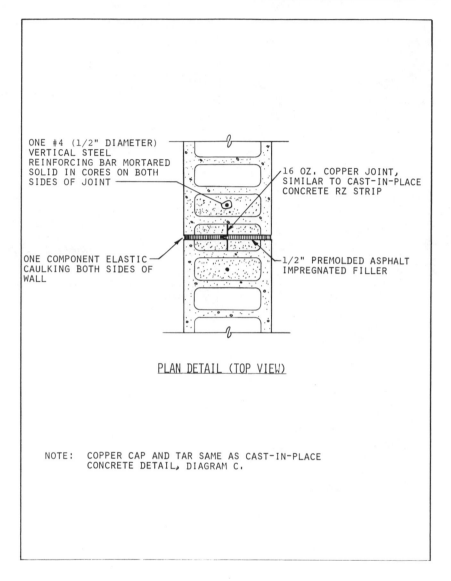

ONE #4 (1/2" DIAMETER) VERTICAL STEEL REINFORCING BAR MORTARED SOLID IN CORES ON BOTH SIDES OF JOINT

16 OZ. COPPER JOINT, SIMILAR TO CAST-IN-PLACE CONCRETE RZ STRIP

ONE COMPONENT ELASTIC CAULKING BOTH SIDES OF WALL

1/2" PREMOLDED ASPHALT IMPREGNATED FILLER

PLAN DETAIL (TOP VIEW)

NOTE: COPPER CAP AND TAR SAME AS CAST-IN-PLACE
        CONCRETE DETAIL, DIAGRAM C.

In a concrete-block wall, viewed from the top in D, blocks are separated by ½-inch asphalt-impregnated fillers, sealed on both the inside and outside of the wall with heavy strips of one-component elastic caulking. As in the poured wall, the copper strip runs vertically to the top of the wall and is sealed by coal tar and a copper cap. For strength, adjacent cores should be filled with reinforced concrete. Joints should appear at least once every twenty-five feet.

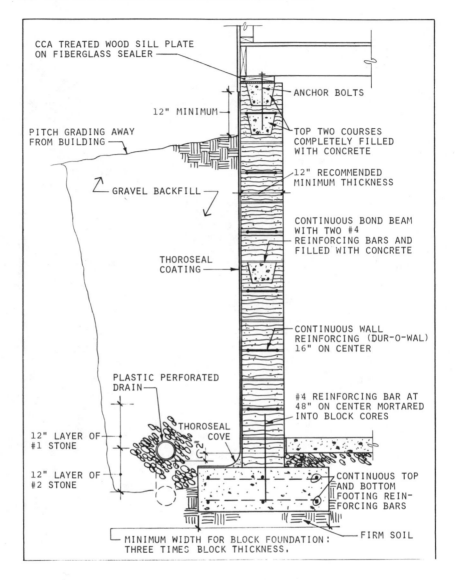

CCA TREATED WOOD SILL PLATE
ON FIBERGLASS SEALER

ANCHOR BOLTS

12" MINIMUM

TOP TWO COURSES
COMPLETELY FILLED
WITH CONCRETE

PITCH GRADING AWAY
FROM BUILDING

12" RECOMMENDED
MINIMUM THICKNESS

GRAVEL BACKFILL

CONTINUOUS BOND BEAM
WITH TWO #4
REINFORCING BARS AND
FILLED WITH CONCRETE

THOROSEAL
COATING

CONTINUOUS WALL
REINFORCING (DUR-O-WAL)
16" ON CENTER

PLASTIC PERFORATED
DRAIN

#4 REINFORCING BAR AT
48" ON CENTER MORTARED
INTO BLOCK CORES

THOROSEAL
COVE

12" LAYER OF
#1 STONE

2"

12" LAYER OF
#2 STONE

CONTINUOUS TOP
AND BOTTOM
FOOTING REIN-
FORCING BARS

FIRM SOIL

MINIMUM WIDTH FOR BLOCK FOUNDATION:
THREE TIMES BLOCK THICKNESS.

DIAGRAM 6 (A & B):

BLOCK-WALL cross section shows construction differing from the conventional in two major respects: It includes *bond beams,* layers of concrete strengthened with two continuous reinforcing bars, and it employs solid rather than hollow blocks for the top two courses.

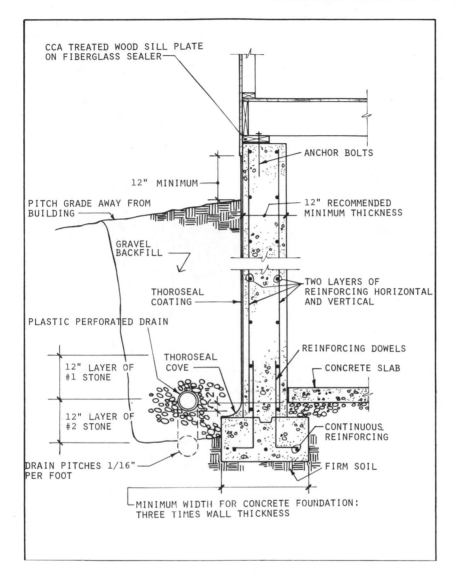

CCA TREATED WOOD SILL PLATE
ON FIBERGLASS SEALER

ANCHOR BOLTS

12" MINIMUM

PITCH GRADE AWAY FROM
BUILDING

12" RECOMMENDED
MINIMUM THICKNESS

GRAVEL
BACKFILL

THOROSEAL
COATING

TWO LAYERS OF
REINFORCING HORIZONTAL
AND VERTICAL

PLASTIC PERFORATED DRAIN

THOROSEAL
COVE

REINFORCING DOWELS

CONCRETE SLAB

12" LAYER OF
#1 STONE

12" LAYER OF
#2 STONE

CONTINUOUS
REINFORCING

DRAIN PITCHES 1/16"
PER FOOT

FIRM SOIL

MINIMUM WIDTH FOR CONCRETE FOUNDATION:
THREE TIMES WALL THICKNESS

CAST-IN-PLACE FOUNDATION WALL is topped by a sill plate of CCA pressure-treated wood; all lumber that is in close proximity to the earth should be treated. Wall footings are required to be at least twice the width of the wall. Drain should rest atop twelve inches of No. 2 crushed stone, and be covered with another twelve inches of No. 1 crushed stone.

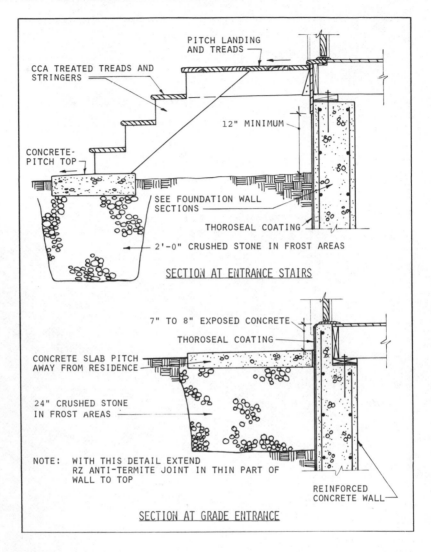

PITCH LANDING
AND TREADS

CCA TREATED TREADS AND
STRINGERS

12" MINIMUM

CONCRETE-
PITCH TOP

SEE FOUNDATION WALL
SECTIONS

THOROSEAL COATING

2'-0" CRUSHED STONE IN FROST AREAS

SECTION AT ENTRANCE STAIRS

7" TO 8" EXPOSED CONCRETE

THOROSEAL COATING

CONCRETE SLAB PITCH
AWAY FROM RESIDENCE

24" CRUSHED STONE
IN FROST AREAS

NOTE: WITH THIS DETAIL EXTEND
RZ ANTI-TERMITE JOINT IN THIN PART OF
WALL TO TOP

REINFORCED
CONCRETE WALL

SECTION AT GRADE ENTRANCE

DIAGRAM 7 (A & B):

ENTRANCE STAIRS, of CCA-treated anti-termite lumber, should rest on a concrete slab; whole stairway unit is sloped away from house to assist runoff. The entire foundation is coated with Thoroseal, including the twelve-inch section shown in diagram to be above grade.

GROUND-LEVEL ENTRANCE ordinarily requires a seven- or eight-inch rise of exposed concrete coated with Thoroseal. Again, concrete entrance slab slopes away from residence.

Appendix C
Manufacturers' List

The following list cites manufacturers used in the development and building of the hazard-free house.

Foundation vents
Riesner Vent Brick Corp.
28–10 38th Ave.
Long Island City, NY 11101

Thoroseal foundation coating
Standard Dry Wall Products
7800 N.W. 38th St.
Miami, FL 33166

*Floor adhesive (Gulf Flooring
    Adhesive [FGC])*
Gulf Adhesive and Resins
616 Markley St.
Norristown, PA 19401

Floor and roof trusses
Trus-Joist Co.
200 Colomet Drive
Delaware, OH 43015

Sill plate sealer (fiberglass)
Johns Manville
Greenwood Plaza
Denver, CO 80217

Roof vents
Bristol Fiberlite Industries,
    Inc.
3200 S. Halladay St.
Santa Ana, CA 92705

*Colored masonry grout for
    exterior block or brick*
Medusa Portland Cement Co.
P.O. Box 5668
Cleveland, OH 44101

Exterior caulking
Sonolastic NP I or NP II (both
    polyurethane)
Sonneborn—Building Products
    Division
Division of Contech, Inc.
7711 Computer Ave.
Minneapolis, MN 55435

Glass sliding doors
Miller Industries
16295 N.W. 13th Ave.
Miami, FL 33169

*Plastic window glazing
transparent to ultraviolet
light (type: Plexiglas II
UVT)*
Rohm & Haas
Philadelphia, PA

Colored grout for interior tile
Hydromet Joint Filler
Upco Co.
Bostik Chemical Group
USM Corp.
4805 Lexington Ave.
Cleveland, OH 44103

*Townsend solid hardwood
prefinished wall plank
paneling*
Townsend Co.
Div. of Pottlatch Corp.
Wood Products
P.O. Box 916
Stuttgart, AR 72160

Hardwood floors
A. Harris Mfg. Co.
   773 East Walnut St.
   Johnson City, TN 37601
B. Memphis Hardwood
   Flooring Co.
   P.O. Box 7253
   Memphis TN 38107

Floor tile adhesive (waterbased)
Chicago Mastic Co.
7100 North Mannheim Rd.
Rosement, Il 60018

*Stain and polyurethane floor
finish*
Dura Seal
Minwax Co., Inc.
72 Oak St.
Clifton, NJ 07014

Vacuum system (built-in)
Vacu-Maid
P.O. Box 1708
Ponca City, OK 74601

*Vacuum cleaner (not built-in;
water type)*
"The Rainbow"
Rexair Inc.
900 Tower Drive, Suite 700
P.O. Box 3610
Troy, MI 48095

Filtration devices:
A. —particles, gases
   —home (and auto)
   —portable, stationary
   Air Conditioning
   Engineers
   P.O. Box 616
   Decatur, IL 62525
B. —particles
   —portable; for insertion
      into ductwork
   Delta Filter Corp.
   Northway 10 Industrial
   Park
   P.O. Box 410
   Clifton Park, NY 12065
C. —particles, gases
   —portable, stationary
   Cleanaire
   P.O. Box 122
   Oak Lawn, IL 60453
D. —particles
   —portable
   Hepanaire HP50
   Dome Laboratories
   Div. of Miles
   Laboratories, Inc.
   West Haven, CT 06516

   Dexon Prime-Aire
   Dexon, Inc.
   3440 Belt Line Blvd.
   Minneapolis, MN 55416

Charcoal filter
—gases
Barnaby-Cheney
Cassady at Eighth Ave.
Columbus, OH 43219

Humidifier (individual room unit)
Vapor-All Brand, mfg. by:
West Bend Co.
West Bend, WI 53095

Humidifier (system)
Model #MA-315
Humid-Aire Corp.
3845 Carnation
Franklin Park, IL 60131

Fireplace
Wells Fireplace Furnaces
3930 West Ajo Way
P.O. Box 7097
Tucson, AZ 85725

Fireplace doors (partially airtight)
Diamond W Products, Inc.
Salina Drive
Colonie
Albany, NY 12205

Rug cleaning
Orvus Extra Granules
Orvus NWA Paste
Procter and Gamble
Cincinnati, OH 45200

Wooden bed (no metal)
Lattoflex Co., Inc.
150 East 58th St.
New York, NY 10022

Dustproof encasings (for mattresses, box springs, pillows)
A. Allergy Free Products for the Homes, Inc.
1162 West Lynn
Springfield, MO 65801
B. Allergens Proof Encasings, Inc.
4046 Superior Ave.
Cleveland, OH 44103

Sauna oven
Nippa Co.
Bruce Crossing
MI 49912

Sauna (nonresinous wood)
Micro Metals, Inc.
10000 Levee St.
P.O. Box 192
Red Wing, MN 55055

Water-source heat pumps
Vaughn Corporation
386 Elm St.
Salisbury, MA 01950

Notes

INTRODUCTION

1. "On the Record," *Time,* 12 June 1978, p. 65.
2. See Malcolm W. Browne, "Chemical Abstracts List World Elements," *New York Times,* 1 January 1978, p. 22; and Barbara J. Culliton, "Toxic Substances Legislation: How Well Are Laws being Implemented?" *Science,* 29 September 1978, p. 1198.
3. "Puzzling Out Man's Ascent," *Time,* 7 November 1977, p. 69.

CHAPTER 1

1. Walter Alvarez, "Food Sensitiveness Can Dull the Brain," *Modern Medicine* 35, no. 6 (13 March 1967): 106.
2. *The Medical Letter* 28, no. 18 (27 August 1976): 120.
3. John Cairns, "The Cancer Problem," *Scientific American,* November 1975, pp. 64–72.
4. "Indoor Smog," *Newsweek,* 30 May 1977, p. 78.
5. Ralph Binder et al., "Importance of the Indoor Environment in Air Pollution Exposure," *Archives of Environmental Health* 31, no. 6 (November–December 1976): 277–79.
6. Gilbert D. Barkin, "Your Health—Allergies," *Today's Education* 59, no. 8 (November 1970): 42.
7. Donald G. McKaba, "Our Purpose," *Allergy and Clinical Immunology News* 1, no. 1 (1979): 1.
8. Richard Mackarness, *Not All in the Mind* (London: Pan, 1976), p. 142.
9. *Human Nature* 1, no. 1 (January 1978): 13.

CHAPTER 2

1. B. Humphrey, "Achew! The Perils of Housedust," *Today's Health*, April 1968, pp. 13–15.
2. G. W. Wharton, "Mites and Commercial Extracts of House Dust," *Science*, 6 March 1970, pp. 1382–83.
3. Lawrence Galton, "Do You Have a Hidden Allergy?" *Popular Science*, August 1960, pp. 86–89.
4. Frank L. Rosen, "The Role of the Allergist in the Battle Against Air Pollution," *Consumer Bulletin* 46 (September 1963): 36–38.
5. Theron G. Randolph, *Human Ecology and Susceptibility to the Chemical Environment* (Springfield, Ill.: Charles C. Thomas, 1962), p. 8.
6. Richard Mackarness, *Not All in the Mind* (London: Pan, 1976), p. 140.
7. Letter from Norman Rafalowsky to editor of *The Daily Freeman*, Kingston, NY, January 8, 1976.

CHAPTER 3

1. See William G. Crook, "The Allergic Tension-Fatigue Syndrome," in F. Speer, ed., *The Allergic Child* (New York: Harper and Row, Hoeber Medical Division, 1963), pp. 229–341; ———, *Can Your Child Read? Is He Hyperactive?* (Jackson, Tenn.; Pedicenter Press, 1975); F. Speer, *Allergy and the Nervous System* (Springfield, Ill.: Charles C. Thomas, 1970); and K. E. Moyer, *The Psychobiology of Aggression* (New York: Harper and Row, 1976).
2. Theron G. Randolph, *Human Ecology and Susceptibility to the Chemical Environment* (Springfield, Ill.: Charles C. Thomas, 1962), pp. 104–05.
3. Craig Hollowell, R. J. Budnitz, and Gregory Traynor, Lawrence Berkeley Laboratory, University of California at Berkeley (paper prepared under the auspices of the Energy Research and Development Administration and presented at the Fourth International Clean Air Congress, Tokyo, 20 May 1977); updated through correspondence with the authors.
4. Ruth Winter, *The Smell Book: Scents, Sex, and Society* (Philadelphia and New York: J. B. Lippincott, 1976), p. 17.
5. Randolph, *Human Ecology*, pp. 41–42.
6. See Ronald J. Young et al., "Benzene in Consumer Products," *Science*, 13 January 1978, p. 248; and "Benzene Dangers in the Home," *Science News*, 8 October 1977, p. 233.
7. S. M. Wolfe and P. A. Greene, petition to S. J. Byington, chairman, Consumer Product Safety Commission, Health Research Group, Washington, D.C., 5 May 1977.
8. Richard D. Steward and Carl L. Hake, "Paint Remover Haz-

ard," *Journal of the American Medical Association* 235, no. 4 (January 1976): 398.

9. Randolph, *Human Ecology*, p. 105.

CHAPTER 4

1. Robert H. Moser, "Ruminations: The Great Winds of the Earth," *Journal of the American Medical Association* 227, no. 2 (14 January 1974): 195–96.

2. See Lewis R. Koller, "Ionization of the Atmosphere and Its Biological Effects," *Journal of The Franklin Institute* 214, no. 5 (November 1932): 555–56; J. A. Crowther, *Ions, Electrons and Ionizing Radiations* (London: Arnold, 1938); J. C. Beckett, "Air Ionization as an Environment Factor," *Electrical Engineering* 73, no. 10 (1954): 916–20; T. L. Martin, "Climate Control Through Ionization," *Journal of The Franklin Institute* 267 (1952): 267–80; and C. P. Yaglou and L. C. Benjamin, "Diurnal and Seasonal Variation in the Small Ion Content of Outdoor and Indoor Air," *Heating, Piping and Air-Conditioning* 6, no. 1 (1934): 25–32.

3. Arnold L. Lieber and Carolyn R. Sherin, "Homicides and the Lunar Cycle: Toward a Theory of Lunar Influence on Human Emotional Disturbance," *American Journal of Psychiatry* 129, no. 1 (July 1972): 69–74.

4. See A. P. Krueger et al., "The Action of Air Ions on Bacteria," *Journal of General Physiology* 41, no. 2 (1957), pp. 359–81; A. P. Krueger et al., "The Biological Mechanisms of Air Ion Action," *Journal of General Physiology* (1957); and A. P. Krueger, "Are Negative Air Ions Good For You?" *The New Scientist* 58, no. 850 (14 June 1973), pp. 668–70.

5. Fred Soyka with Alan Edmonds, *The Ion Effect: How Air Electricity Rules Your Life and Health* (New York: E. P. Dutton, 1977), p. 33.

6. See F. G. Sulman, "Effects of Hot Dry Desert Winds (Sharav, Hamsin) on the Metabolism of Hormones," *Journal of the Medical Association of Israel* 63, no. 1 (July 1962): 133; "Urinalysis of Patients Suffering from Climatic Heat Stress (Sharav)," *International Journal of Biometeorology* 14, no. 1 (1970): 45–53; "Serotonin-Migraine in Climatic Heat Stress: Its Prophylaxis and Treatment" (paper delivered at the International Headache Symposium, Elsinore, Denmark, 1971), pp. 205–10; and "Adrenal Medullary Exhaustion from Tropical Winds and Its Management," *Israel Journal of Medical Sciences* 9, no. 8 (1973): 1022.

7. Quoted in Robert O'Brien, "Magic Ions in the Air," *The Rotarian* 96, no. 7 (October 1960): 41.

8. E. T. Pierce and A. L. Whitson, "Atmospheric Electricity in a Typical American Bathroom," *Weather* 21, no. 12 (December 1966): 449–55.

9. E. A. Mortimer, R. R. Monson, and B. MacMahon, "Reduction in Mortality from Coronary Heart Disease in Men Residing at High

Altitudes," *New England Journal of Medicine* 296, no. 11 (17 March 1977): 581–86.

10. B. Maczysnki, "Effect of the Presence of Man on the Air Ion Density in an Office Room," *International Journal of Biometeorology* 15, no. 1 (1971): 11–24.

11. John C. Beckett, in *Journal of American Society of Heating, Refrigeration and Air-Conditioning* 1: 47.

12. T. L. Martin, "Climate Control Through Ionization," *Journal of The Franklin Institute* 254 (1952): 267–80.

13. C. W. Hansell, "An Attempt to Define 'Ionization of the Air' " (Proceedings of the International Conference on Ionization of the Air, Philadelphia, 1961).

14. See A. P. Krueger, "Preliminary Consideration of the Biological Significance of Air Ions," *Scientia* 104 (September-October 1969): 8; "The Action of Air Ions on Bacteria," *Journal of General Physiology* (University of California, Berkeley, 1957); "The Biological Properties of Gaseous Ions," *Encyclopedia of Science and Technology* (New York: McGraw-Hill, 1962); "Air Ion Effects on the Iron Metabolism of Barley," *Proceedings of the Botanical Society* (Japan, 1965); "Small Air Ions: Their Effect on Blood Levels of Serotonin in Terms of Modern Physical Theory," *International Journal of Biometeorology* 12, no. 103 (July 1968): 225; and "The Influence of Air Ions on a Model of Respiratory Disease," *Proceedings of the World Congress of Medicine and Biology of the Environment* (Paris: 1974).

15. Soyka, *The Ion Effect*, p. 33.

16. O'Brien, "Magic Ions in the Air," p. 63.

CHAPTER 5

1. F. A. Brown, "The 'Clock' Timing Biological Rhythms," *American Scientist* 60, no. 6 (December 1972): 756.

2. Robert O. Becker, testimony before the State of New York Public Service Commission (Cases 26529 and 26559), "Hearings on Health and Safety of 765-KV Transmission Lines."

3. Ibid. and J. A. Spadero, "Electrical Stimulation of Partial Limb Generation in Mammals," *Bulletin of the New York Academy of Medicine* 48, 2d ser. (1972): 624.

4. H. Friedman and R. O. Becker, "Geomagnetic Parameters and Psychiatric Hospital Admissions," *Nature* 200 (1963): 626.

5. Robert O. Becker, "Electromagnetic Forces and Life Processes," *Technology Review* 75, no. 2 (December 1972).

6. Robert O. Becker, "The Significance of Bioelectric Potentials," *Bioelectrochemistry and Bioenergetics* 1 (1974): 187–99; and "Magnetic Man," *Newsweek*, 13 May 1963, pp. 90–91.

7. See A. P. Krueger, "Preliminary Consideration of the Biological Significance of Air Ions," *Scientia* 104 (September-October 1969): 8; A. P. Kreuger, S. Kotaka, and P. C. Andriese, "The Effect of Abnormally Low Concentrations of Air Ions on the Growth of *Hordenum Vulgaris*," *International Journal of Biometeorology* 9 (1965): 201–

09; and Chr. Bach, *Ions for Breathing: Control of the Air-electrical Climate for Health* (Oxford and London: Pergamon Press, 1967), p. 68.

8. A. P. Krueger and E. J. Reed, "Biological Impact of Small Air Ions," *Science*, 24 September 1976, pp. 1208–13.

9. A. P. Dubrov, *The Geomagnetic Field and Life*, trans. Frank L. Sinclair (New York: Plenum Press, 1978), p. 42.

10. Ibid., p. 44.

11. Cited in "GAO: Low Microwave Levels May Harm," *Science News*, 22 April 1978, p. 247.

12. Quoted in Peter Gwynne, "The Flap over the Zap," *Newsweek*, 17 July 1978, p. 89.

13. "Are Americans Being Zapped?" *Time*, 28 August 1978, p. 43.

14. Paul Brodeur, "Microwaves," *New Yorker*, 13 December 1976, pp. 50–57, and 20 December 1976, pp. 43–44.

15. James L. Breeling, "Effectiveness and Hazards of Microwave Cooking," *Journal of the American Medical Association* 213, no. 4 (27 July 1970): 663.

16. *U.S. Naval Bulletin*, July 1943.

17. Frederic G. Hirsh and John T. Parker, "Bilateral Lenticular Opacities Occurring in a Technician Operating a Microwave Generator," *Archives of Industrial Hygiene and Occupational Medicine* 6 (December 1952): 512–17.

18. See D. Dodge and S. Kassel, "Soviet Research on the Neural Effects of Microwaves," Aerospace Technology Division, Library of Congress, Washington, D.C., 1966; and A. S. Presman, *Electromagnetic Fields and Life* (Moscow: Izd-Ro-Nauka, 1968), p. 288.

19. Brodeur, "Microwaves," *New Yorker*, 13 December 1976.

20. John H. Heller, in correspondence with the author, 24 October 1978; see G. H. Mickey, "Electromagnetism and Its Effect on the Organism," *New York State Journal of Medicine* (July 1963); and John H. Heller, "Cellular Effect of Microwave Radiation" (presented at the Symposium on the Biological Effects and Health Implications of Microwave Radiation at the Medical College of Virginia, Richmond, September 1969).

21. Quoted in Peter Gwynne, "The Flap over the Zap," p. 89.

22. Becker, testimony before the State of New York, pp. 4–5.

23. Allan H. Frey et al., "Neural Function and Behavior: Defining a Relationship," *New York Academy of Science Annals* 247 (28 February 1975): 433–39.

24. Clarence W. Wieska, "Human Sensitivity to Electric Fields," *Biomedical Sciences Instrumentation* 1 (1963): 467–74.

CHAPTER 6

1. Fred Soyka with Alan Edmonds, *The Ion Effect: How Air Electricity Rules Your Life and Health* (New York: E. P. Dutton, 1977), pp. 128–29.

2. Robert Gannon, "The Hazards That Surround Us," in *Pennsylvania Burning: Report to the Commonwealth of Pennsylvania from the Governor's Commission on Fire Prevention and Control* (Harrisburg: Pennsylvania Department of Labor, 1976), pp. 186–87.

CHAPTER 7

1. "Chemicals: How Many are There?" *Science*, 13 January 1978, p. 162.

2. Theron G. Randolph, *Human Ecology and Susceptibility to the Chemical Environment* (Springfield, Ill.: Charles C. Thomas, 1962), p. 43.

3. Harvey Foerster, "Merthiolate as an Ixodidicide," *The Schoch Letter* 28, no. 8 (August 1978): 16.

4. See Jack McDowell, *Sunset Ideas for Japanese Gardens* (Menlo Park, Calif.: Lane Books, 1968); K. Asano and G. Takakuwa, *Invitation to Japanese Gardens* (Rutland, Vt.: Charles Tuttle, 1970); and J. I. Rodale and Glen Johns, *Lawn Beauty the Organic Way* (Emmaus, Pa.: Rodale Books, 1970).

5. Jerome Olds, *The Encyclopedia of Organic Farming* (Emmaus, Pa.: Rodale Rooks, 1959).

CHAPTER 8

1. Quoted in Frank L. Rosen, "The Role of the Allergist in the Battle Against Air Pollution," *Consumer Bulletin*, September 1963, pp. 36–38.

2. L. Koller, "Ionization of the Atmosphere and Its Iological Biological Effects," *Journal of The Franklin Institute* 214, no. 5 (November 1932): 543–68.

3. Rosen, "The Role of the Allergist."

4. E. A. Mortimer, R. R. Monson, and B. MacMahon, "Reduction in Mortality from Coronary Heart Disease in Men Residing at High Altitudes," *New England Journal of Medicine* 296, no. 11 (17 March 1977): 15–20.

5. Theron G. Randolph, *Human Ecology and Susceptibility to the Chemical Environment* (Springfield, Ill.: Charles C. Thomas, 1962), p. 48.

6. Theron G. Randolph, excerpted from speech reprinted in *Human Ecology Study Group Bulletin*, Summer 1977.

7. Thomas J. Mason, *Atlas of Cancer Mortality for U.S. Counties: 1950–1969* (Washington, D.C.: National Cancer Institute, 1975).

8. "The Greening of Arizona," *Time*, 3 September 1973, p. 81.

9. Mortimer et al., "Reduction in Mortality."

10. "Community Water Supply Study: Significance of National Findings," U.S. Department of Health, Education, and Welfare, Public Health Service, July 1970, p. 7.

11. Quoted in James McDermott, "Future Program of the Bureau of Water Hygiene" (paper presented at the 50th Anniversary Meeting

of the Conference of State Sanitary Engineers, Minneapolis, 26 May 1970), p. 1.

12. Quoted in David Zwick and Marcy Benstock, *Water Wasteland* (New York: Bantam Books, 1972), p. 7.

13. Cited in "The River Still Gets Chemicals," Kingston, N.Y., *Daily Freeman*, 28 September 1977, p. 1.

14. Samuel H. Watson and Charles S. Kibler, "Drinking Water as a Cause of Asthma," *Journal of Allergy* 5, no. 1 (1934): 197.

15. J. Chen and G. Smith, "Mechanisms of Catalytic and Sonocatalytic Oxidation in Waste Water Treatment" (paper presented at the 172d ACS National Meeting, San Francisco, 29 August 1976).

16. Robert H. Harris and Edward M. Brecher, "Is the Water Safe to Drink?" Collected reprints from *Consumer Reports*, 1974, p. 10.

17. R. D. Zielhus, "Interrelationship of Biochemical Responses to the Absorption of Inorganic Lead," *Archives of Environmental Health* 23, no. 4 (October 1971): 299–311.

18. See H. A. Schroeder, "Relation Between Mortality from Cardiovascular Disease and Treated Water Supplies," *Journal of the American Medical Association* 172, no. 17 (23 April 1960): 1902–8; and H. A. Schroeder and J. Buckman, "Cadmium Hypertension: Its Reversal in Rats by Zinc Chelate," *Archives of Environmental Health* 14, no. 5 (May 1967): 693–97.

19. L. Koller, J. Exon, and J. Roan, "Antibody Suppression by Cadmium," *Archives of Environmental Health* 30, no. 12 (December 1975): 598–601.

20. H. A. Schroeder, *The Poisons Around Us* (Bloomington: Indiana University Press, 1974), p. 89.

21. See A. Prasad, *Zinc Metabolism* (Springfield, Ill.: Charles C. Thomas, 1966), pp. 38–39; J. Parizek and I. Ostadalova, "The Protective Effects of Small Amounts of Selenite on Sublimate Intoxication," *Experientia* 23 (1967): 142–43; H. E. Ganther and C. A. Baumann, "Selenium Metabolism: Effects of Diet, Arsenic and Cadmium," *Journal of Nutrition* 77 (1962): 210–16; R. J. Shamberger and C. E. Willis, "Selenium Distribution and Human Cancer Mortality," *Critical Reviews in Laboratory Sciences* 2 (June 1971): 211–21; and R. J. Shamberger, "Relationship of Selenium to Cancer: Inhibiting Effect of Selenium on Carcinogenesis," *Journal of the National Cancer Institute* 44 (April 1970): 931–36.

22. H. A. Schroeder, "Relation Between Mortality from Cardiovascular Disease and Treated Water Supplies," pp. 1902–8.

CHAPTER 9

1. Ken Kern, *The Owner-Built Home* (Oakhurst, Calif., Ken Kern Drafting, 1972), p. iv.

2. Rex Roberts, *Your Engineered House* (New York: M. Evans, 1964), pp. 20–21.

3. Robert Gannon, "Ground-Water Heat Pumps: Heat and Cool from Your Own Well," *Popular Science*, February 1978, pp. 78–82.

4. Ken Gilmore, "Higher Efficiency with Solar-Assisted Heat Pumps," *Popular Science*, May 1978, pp. 86–90.

5. See Kern, *Owner-Built Home*, chapter entitled "Ventilation."

6. *In the Bank . . . or up the Chimney?* Department of Housing and Urban Development, Washington, D.C., April 1975; available from U.S. Government Printing Office, Washington, D.C. 20402, for $1.70 (stock number 023-000-00297-3).

7. "Cellulose Insulation: Proceed with Caution," *Consumer Reports*, February 1970, p. 69.

8. Elliot Richman, "Millions of Homes May Have Toxic Insulation," *Medical Tribune and Medical News* 19, no. 9 (1 March 1978).

9. "Mobile-Home Disease Traced to Formaldehyde," *Medical World News* 19, no. 6 (20 March 1978): 16.

10. Peter Breysse, "Formaldehyde in Mobile and Conventional Homes," *Environmental Health and Safety News* 25, nos. 1–6 (January-June 1977): 1–20.

11. See *Subterranean Termites: Their Prevention and Control in Buildings*, Home and Garden Bulletin No. 64, U.S. Department of Agriculture, 1972, available from the Government Printing Office, Washington, D.C. 20402, for 45 cents (stock number 001-03459-6); and Arnold Mallis, *Handbook of Pest Control*, 5th ed. (New York: MacNair and Durland, 1969).

12. See M. P. Levi et al., "Uptake by Grape Plants of Preservatives from Pressure-Treated Posts Not Detected," *Forest Products Journal* 24, no. 9 (September 1974): 97–98; and R. D. Arsenault, "CCA-Treated Wood Foundations: A Study of Permanence, Effectiveness, Durability, and Environmental Considerations" (paper presented at the Annual Meeting of the American Wood-Preservers' Association, San Francisco, April 1975).

13. Kern, *Owner-Built Home*, pp. 28–29.

14. John Ott, *Health and Light* (Old Greenwich, Conn.: Devin-Adair, 1973).

15. "Com-Ply: Future Frame-Up for Housing," *Popular Science*, June 1976, p. 72.

16. Letter from James M. Sovaiko, Throop, Pa., printed in *Popular Science*, April 1976.

17. Reported by Francis Silver, an engineer in Martinsburg, West Virginia, in the Human Ecology Study Group newsletter (now combined with H.E.A.L.; 505 North Lake Shore Drive, Suite 403, Chicago, IL 60611), February 1976, p. 6.

18. John S. Neuberger, "Formaldehyde Toxicity," Ph.D. thesis, Department of Environmental Medicine, Johns Hopkins University, 22 March 1973, p. 16.

19. "Asbestos in Adhesives: Health Hazard," *Science News*, 16 August 1975, pp. 100–01.

20. Breysse, "Formaldehyde in Mobile and Conventional Homes," *Environmental Health and Safety News* pp. 1–20.

21. R. Siksna, "Positive Ions Formed by an Open Electric Heater," *Arkiz for Fysik* 5, no. 25 (1952): 531–43.

APPENDIX A

1. Theron G. Randolph, *Human Ecology and Susceptibility to the Chemical Environment* (Springfield, Ill.: Charles C. Thomas, 1962), p. 120.

Index